PSYCHIATRIC
DRUG
REACTIONS AND
INTERACTIONS

PSYCHIATRIC
DRUG
REACTIONS AND
INTERACTIONS

JEROME Z. LITT, MD

Assistant Clinical Professor of Dermatology
Case Western Reserve University School of Medicine
Cleveland, Ohio

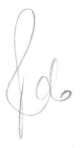

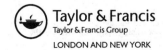

Taylor & Francis
Taylor & Francis Group
LONDON AND NEW YORK

©2005 Taylor & Francis, an imprint of the Taylor & Francis Group

First published in the United Kingdom in 2005
by Taylor & Francis,
an imprint of the Taylor & Francis Group,
2 Park Square, Milton Park
Abingdon, Oxon OX14 4RN, UK

Tel	+44 (0) 20 7017 6000
Fax:	+44 (0) 20 7017 6699
Website:	www.tandf.co.uk

British Library Cataloguing in Publication Data

Data available on application

Library of Congress Cataloguing-in-Publication Data

Data available on application

ISBN 0-415-38379-X

Distributed in North and South America by
Taylor & Francis
2000 NW Corporate Blvd
Boca Raton, FL 33431, USA

Within Continental USA
Tel: 800 272 7737; Fax: 800 374 3401
Outside Continental USA
Tel: 561 994 0555; Fax: 561 361 6018
E-mail: orders@crcpress.com

Distributed in the rest of the world by
Thomson Publishing Services
Cheriton House
North Way
Andover, Hampshire SP10 5BE, UK
Tel: +44 (0) 1264 332424
E-mail: salesorder.tandf@thomsonpublishingservices.co.uk

Composition by AMA DataSet Limited, Preston, UK
Printed and bound by Antony Rowe Ltd., Chippenham, Wiltshire, UK

CONTENTS

INTRODUCTION

Any drug can cause any rash.

According to the World Health Organization, an adverse reaction (ADR) – or adverse event (ADE) – to a drug has been defined as any noxious or unintended reaction to a drug that has been administered in standard doses by the proper route for the purposes of prophylaxis, diagnosis, or treatment. This definition does not include abuse, overdose, withdrawal, or error of administration. While most reactions are mild and self-limited, severe and life-threatening reactions do occur, as seen in Anorexia and Suicidal ideation. Death is the ultimate adverse drug event, and has now been incorporated into the book.

ADRs are underreported and thus are an underestimated cause of morbidity and mortality. The incidence and severity of ADRs can be influenced by age, sex, disease, genetic factors, type of drug, route of administration, duration of therapy, dosage, and bioavailability, as well as interactions with other drugs. It has been estimated that fatal ADRs are the third or fourth leading cause of death in the US.

This Pocketbook of Psychiatric Drug Reactions and Interactions describes and catalogs the adverse effects of **over 170** commonly prescribed and over-the-counter generic drugs and herbals used in psychiatry or having psychiatric side effects. These drugs include classes such as Anticonvulsants, Antidepressants, Antipsychotic agents, Anxiolytics, Sedatives & Hypnotics, Benzodiazepines, Hypnotics, SSRIs, and Tranquilizers. The drugs have been listed and indexed by both their **Generic** and **Trade** (**Brand**) names for easy accessibility.

In addition to adverse drug reactions, there are many severe, hazardous **interactions** between two or more drugs. I have incorporated only the clinically important, potentially hazardous drug interactions that can trigger potential harm, and could be life-threatening. These interactions are predictable and well documented in controlled studies; they should be avoided.

For each drug, I have listed the known adverse side effects – in the form of drug reactions – that can develop from the use of the corresponding drug. These include those involving the skin, hair, nails, cardiologic, eyes, hematopoietic and mucous membrane side effects. The section entitled 'other' includes such reactions as tinnitus, serotonin syndrome, depression, rhabdomyolysis, insomnia, and death.

The first part of the book lists, in alphabetical order, the **Generic** and **Trade** name drugs with their corresponding names for easy access to the **A-Z** section – the main body of the book. Next comes a listing of the various **Classes** of drugs, and those **Generic** drugs that belong to each class. The last part of the book includes listings of common psychiatric reactions caused mainly by non-psychiatric drugs.

The major portion of the Pocketbook – the body of the work – lists the Generic drugs, herbals and supplements in alphabetical order and the adverse reactions that can arise from their use. The numbers in square brackets refer to the number of references recorded for each reaction. These references are available on my website (www.drugeruptiondata.com) or in the latest edition of the Drug Eruption Reference Manual.

USAGE, STYLE & CONVENTIONS EMPLOYED IN THIS POCKETBOOK

The **Generic Drug** name is at the top of each page.

The **Trade (Brand) Name(s)** are then listed alphabetically. When there are many **Trade Names**, the ten (or so) most commonly recognized ones are listed. This compilation lists and cross-references both the **Trade *and* Generic** names of all the cataloged drugs. Following the more common **Trade Name** drugs are recorded – in parentheses – the latest name of the pharmaceutical company that is marketing the drug.

Beneath the **Trade Name** listing is a list of Other **Common Trade Names**, those drugs from other countries. Then appear the **Indication(s)**, the **Category** in which the drug belongs, and the **Half-Life** of each drug, when known, and the **Potentially hazardous interactions** between drugs. On occasion, an important or pertinent **Note** will follow.

Reactions: These are the **Adverse Reactions** to the particular **Generic** drug.

They are classified into **Categories: Skin, Hair, Nails, Hematopoietic, Eyes**, and **Other**. (**Other** refers to **Mucous Membrane, Teeth, Muscle** and various other **Reactions**.) **Reactions** are listed alphabetically under each heading. Alongside each **Reaction Pattern** are square bracketed numbers that refer to the number of references in the main Drug Eruption Reference Manual and my website. Numbers in round brackets refer to the incidence of the reaction, e.g. (3 cases) or (15%).

In the case of **herbals** and **supplements**, the format is slightly different. The herbals feature the scientific species and genus, purported indications and other uses. Then follows the same format as the generic drugs.

There are occasions when there are very few adverse reactions to a specific drug. These drugs are still included, since there is often **positive significance in negative findings**.

Jerome Z. Litt, M.D.
June, 2005

INDEX OF GENERIC AND TRADE NAMES

CLASSES OF DRUGS

Anticonvulsants
acetazolamine
amobarbital
carbamazepine
clonazepam
clorazepate
ethosuximide
ethotoin
felbamate
fosphenytoin
gabapentin
lamotrigine
levetiracetam
mephenytoin
mephobarbital
methsuximide
oxcarbazepine
paramethadione
pentobarbital
phenobarbital
phensuximide
phenytoin
primidone
thiopental
tiagabine
topiramate
trimethadione
valproic acid
vigabatrin
zonisamide

Antidepressants
amitriptyline
amoxapine
benactyzine
bupropion
citalopram
clomipramine
desipramine
doxepin
duloxetine
escitalopram
fluoxetine
fluvoxamine
imipramine
isocarboxazid
maprotiline
mirtazapine
nefazodone
nortriptyline
paroxetine
phenelzine
prazepam
protriptyline
sertraline
tranylcypromine
trazodone
trimipramine
venlafaxine

Antipsychotic agents
amitriptyline
aripiprazole
chlorpromazine
clozapine
fluphenazine
haloperidol
lithium
loxapine
mesoridazine
molindone
olanzapine
perphenazine
pimozide
prochlorperazine
promazine
quetiapine
risperidone
thioridazine
thiothixene
trifluoperazine
ziprasidone

Anxiolytics, Sedatives & Hypnotics
alprazolam
amitriptyline
amobarbital
aprobarbital
buspirone
butabarbital
butalbital
chloral hydrate
chlordiazepoxide
chlormezanone
clonazepam
clorazepate
dexmedetomidine
diazepam
droperidol

doxepin
estazolam
ethchlorvynol
flurazepam
hydroxyzine
kava
ketamine
lavender
lemon balm
lorazepam
mephobarbital
meprobamate
mesoridazine
midazolam
oxazepam
paroxetine
pentazocine
pentobarbital
phenobarbital
prazepam
prochlorperazine
propofol
quazepam
secobarbital
sertraline
temazepam
thiopental
triazolam
trifluoperazine
tryptophan
valerian
venlafaxine
zaleplon
zolpidem

Benzodiazepines
alprazolam
amitriptyline
chlordiazepoxide
clonazepam
clorazepate
diazepam
estazolam
flurazepam
lorazepam
midazolam
oxazepam
prazepam
quazepam
temazepam
triazolam

Hypnotics
amobarbital

butalbital
chloral hydrate
chlordiazepoxide
estazolam
ethchlorvynol
flurazepam
ketamine
midazolam
oxazepam
pentobarbital
phenobarbital
prazepam
quazepam
secobarbital
temazepam
triazolam
valerian
zaleplon
zolpidem

SSRIs
citalopram
duloxetine
escitalopram
fluoxetine
fluvoxamine
paroxetine
sertraline
venlafaxine

Tranquilizers
buspirone
chlordiazepoxide
chlormezanone
chlorpromazine
clorazepate
diazepam
doxepin
fluphenazine
haloperidol
hydroxyzine
lorazepam
loxapine
meprobamate
molindone
oxazepam
pimozide
prochlorperazine
promazine
promethazine
reserpine
St John's wort
trifluoperazine
trimeprazine

ACAMPROSATE

Trade names: Aotal; Campral (Forest) (Lipha)
Indications: Alcohol dependence
Category: Antialcoholic
Half-life: 20–33 hours

Reactions

Skin

Abscess (<1%)
Acne (<1%)
Allergic reactions (sic) (<1%)
Chills (>1%)
Diaphoresis (2%)
Eczema (<1%)
Erythema
Erythema multiforme [1]
Exanthems (<1%)
Exfoliative dermatitis (<1%)
Facial edema (<0.1%)
Flu-like syndrome (>1%)
Peripheral edema (>1%)
Photosensitivity (<0.1%)
Pruritus (4%) [1]
Rash (sic) (>1%)
Urticaria (<1%)
Vesiculobullous eruption (<1%)
Xerosis (<1%)

Hair

Hair – alopecia

Eyes

Amblyopia (<1%)
Diplopia (<1%)
Ophthalmitis (<0.1%)
Photophobia (<0.1%)

Hematopoietic

Ecchymoses (<1%)
Thrombocytopenia (<1%)

Cardiovascular

Chest pain (>1%)

Other

Abdominal pain (>1%)

Anxiety (6%)
Arthralgia (>1%)
Asthenia (6%)
Back pain (>1%)
Bronchitis (>1%)
Cough (>1%)
Death (<0.1%)
Depression (5%)
Dizziness (3%)
Dysgeusia (>1%)
Dysphagia (<1%)
Fever (<1%)
Headache (>1%)
Infections (sic) (>1%)
Insomnia (7%)
Leg cramps (<1%)
Lymphadenopathy
Myalgia (>1%)
Myopathy (<0.1%)
Oral ulceration (<0.1%)
Pain (3%)
Paresthesias (2%)
Pharyngitis (2%)
Phlebitis (<1%)
Rhinitis (>1%)
Seizures (<1%)
Sialorrhea (<0.1%)
Suicide (attempted) (>1%)
Syncope (>1%)
Tinnitus (<1%)
Tremor (>1%)
Twitching (<0.1%)
Vaginitis (<1%)
Vertigo
Xerostomia (2%)

ALPRAZOLAM

Trade name: Xanax (Pfizer)
Other common trade names: *Alprox; APO-Alpraz; Cassadan; Kalma; Nu-Alprax; Ralozam; Tafil*
Indications: Anxiety, depression, panic attacks
Category: Benzodiazepine anxiolytic
Half-life: 11–16 hours
Clinically important, potentially hazardous interactions with: alcohol, aprepitant, clarithromycin, CNS depressants, delavirdine, digoxin, efavirenz, fluconazole, fluoxetine, fluvoxamine, **grapefruit juice**, indinavir, itraconazole, ivermectin, **kava**, ketoconazole, propoxyphene, ritonavir, saquinavir, **St John's wort**, telithromycin

---

Reactions

Skin
 Acne [1]
 Allergic reactions (sic) [1]
 Dermatitis (3.8%) [5]
 Diaphoresis (15.8%)
 Edema (4.9%)
 Exanthems [1]
 Photosensitivity [4]
 Phototoxicity [2]
 Pruritus [2]
 Purpura
 Rash (sic) (10.8%) [4]
 Urticaria
 Xerosis [1]

Other
 Dysgeusia (<1%) [1]
 Galactorrhea
 Gynecomastia
 Headache
 Oral ulceration
 Paresthesias (2.4%)
 Pseudolymphoma [1]
 Seizures [1]
 Sialopenia (32.8%)
 Sialorrhea (4.2%)
 Tinnitus
 Xerostomia (14.7%) [5]

AMITRIPTYLINE

Trade names: Elavil (AstraZeneca); Limbitrol (Valeant)
Other common trade names: *Amineurin; Domical; Laroxyl; Lentizol; Levate; Novotriptyn; Saroten; Tryptanol; Tryptizol*
Indications: Depression
Category: Antimigraine; Tricyclic antidepressant
Half-life: 10–25 hours
Clinically important, potentially hazardous interactions with: amprenavir, clonidine, **ephedra**, epinephrine, **eucalyptus**, guanethidine, isocarboxazid, linezolid, MAO inhibitors, phenelzine, quinolones, sparfloxacin, **St John's wort**, tranylcypromine

Limbitrol is amitriptyline and chlordiazepoxide

Reactions

Skin
Acne
Allergic reactions (sic) (<1%)
Angioedema [1]
Bullous eruption (<1%) [1]
Dermatitis [1]
Dermatitis herpetiformis [1]
Diaphoresis (1–10%) [1]
Edema [1]
Erythema
Erythema annulare centrifugum [1]
Erythroderma [1]
Exanthems
Exfoliative dermatitis
Facial edema
Fixed eruption [1]
Lichen planus [1]
Lupus erythematosus [1]
Necrosis [1]
Petechiae
Photosensitivity (<1%) [3]
Pigmentation [3]
Pruritus [3]
Purpura [2]
Rash (sic)
Urticaria
Vasculitis [1]

Hair
Hair – alopecia (<1%) [1]

Eyes
Nystagmus [1]

Cardiovascular
Congestive heart failure [1]
Flushing
QT prolongation [1]
Torsades de pointes [1]

Other
Ageusia
Anaphylactoid reactions
Black tongue
Bromhidrosis
Depression [1]
Dysgeusia (>10%)
Galactorrhea (<1%)
Glossitis
Gynecomastia (<1%)
Headache
Hypersensitivity [1]
Lymphoid hyperplasia [1]
Oral mucosal eruption [1]
Paresthesias
Parkinsonism
Pseudolymphoma [2]
Rhabdomyolysis [1]
Seizures [1]
Sialopenia [1]
Sialorrhea
Stomatitis [1]

Stomatopyrosis
Tardive dyskinesia [1]
Tinnitus
Tongue edema

Tremor
Vaginitis
Xerostomia (>10%) [4]

AMOBARBITAL

Trade name: Amytal
Other common trade names: *Amytal Sodium; Isoamitil Sedante; Neur-Amyl; Novambarb; Sodium Amytal*
Indications: Insomnia, sedation
Category: Anticonvulsant; Barbiturate sedative-hypnotic
Half-life: initial: 40 minutes; terminal: 20 hours
Clinically important, potentially hazardous interactions with: alcohol, dicumarol, ethanolamine, warfarin

Reactions

Skin
  Acne
  Angioedema
  Bullous eruption
  Erythema [1]
  Exanthems
  Exfoliative dermatitis (<1%)
  Photosensitivity
  Purpura
  Rash (sic) (<1%)
  Stevens–Johnson syndrome (<1%)

  Toxic epidermal necrolysis [1]
  Urticaria (<1%)

Other
  Headache
  Hypersensitivity
  Injection-site pain (>10%)
  Rhabdomyolysis [1]
  Serum sickness
  Thrombophlebitis (<1%)

AMOXAPINE

Trade name: Amoxapine (Watson)
Other common trade names: *Amoxan; Asendis; Defanyl; Demolox*
Indications: Depression
Category: Tricyclic antidepressant
Half-life: 11–30 hours
Clinically important, potentially hazardous interactions with: amprenavir, clonidine, epinephrine, guanethidine, isocarboxazid, linezolid, MAO inhibitors, phenelzine, quinolones, sparfloxacin, tranylcypromine

Reactions

Skin
  Acne

Acute generalized exanthematous
  pustulosis (AGEP) [3]

Allergic reactions (sic) (<1%)
Dermatitis
Diaphoresis (1–10%)
Edema (>1%)
Erythema multiforme (observation) [1]
Exanthems [2]
Neuroleptic malignant syndrome [1]
Neutrophilic dermatosis [1]
Petechiae
Photosensitivity (<1%)
Pruritus (<1%) [1]
Purpura
Rash (sic) (>1%)
Side effects (sic) (5.1%) [1]
Toxic epidermal necrolysis [2]
Urticaria (<1%)
Vasculitis (<1%) [1]
Xerosis

Hair
Hair – alopecia (<1%)

Cardiovascular
Flushing

Other
Adult respiratory distress syndrome (ARDS) [1]
Black tongue
Bromhidrosis
Dysgeusia (>10%)
Galactorrhea (<1%) [2]
Glossitis
Gynecomastia (<1%)
Headache
Paresthesias (<1%)
Pseudoparkinsonism
Sialorrhea
Stomatitis
Tinnitus
Tremor
Vaginitis
Xerostomia (14%) [1]

APROBARBITAL

Trade name: Alurate (Roche)
Indications: Short-term sedation, sleep induction
Category: Barbiturate
Half-life: 14–34 hours
Clinically important, potentially hazardous interactions with: alcohol, brompheniramine, buclizine, dicumarol, ethanolamine, warfarin

Reactions

Skin
Angioedema
Exanthems
Exfoliative dermatitis
Purpura
Rash (sic)

Stevens–Johnson syndrome
Urticaria

Other
Rhabdomyolysis [1]
Serum sickness

ARIPIPRAZOLE

Trade name: Abilify (Bristol-Myers Squibb)
Other common trade name: *Abilitat*
Indications: Schizophrenia
Category: Antipsychotic
Half-life: 75–94 hours
Clinically important, potentially hazardous interactions with: carbamazepine, ketoconazole, quinidine

Reactions

Skin
  Acne
  Candidiasis
  Cheilitis
  Chills
  Diaphoresis
  Eczema
  Exanthems
  Exfoliative dermatitis
  Flu-like syndrome
  Neuroleptic malignant syndrome
  Peripheral edema
  Pruritus
  Psoriasis
  Rash (sic) (6%)
  Seborrhea
  Ulcerations
  Upper respiratory infection
  Urticaria
  Vesiculobullous eruption
  Xerosis

Hair
  Hair – alopecia

Eyes
  Blepharitis
  Lacrimation
  Xerophthalmia

Cardiovascular
  ECG changes (abnormalities) [1]

Other
  Akathisia (10%) [1]
  Anxiety (15%)

Arthralgia
Bone or joint pain
Cough (3%)
Depression
Dysgeusia
Fever (2%)
Gingival hemorrhage
Gingivitis
Glossitis
Gynecomastia
Headache
Hiccups
Hyperesthesia
Mastodynia
Myalgia
Myasthenia
Oral candidiasis
Oral ulceration
Oral vesiculation
Phlebitis
Priapism
Rhabdomyolysis
Seizures
Sialorrhea
Stomatitis
Tendinitis
Thrombophlebitis
Tinnitus
Tongue edema
Tremor (3%)
Twitching
Vulvovaginal candidiasis
Xerostomia

BENACTYZINE

Trade name: Deprol
Indications: Depression, anxiety
Category: Antidepressant
Half-life: N/A

Deprol is benactyzine and meprobamate

Note: Most of the adverse reactions are due to meprobamate (which see)

Reactions

Skin
Angioedema
Bullous eruption
Edema
Erythema multiforme
Exanthems [1]
Exfoliative dermatitis
Fixed eruption
Petechiae
Pruritus
Urticaria

Hematopoietic
Ecchymoses

Other
Anaphylactoid reactions
Paresthesias
Stomatitis
Xerostomia

BENZPHETAMINE

Trade name: Didrex (Pfizer)
Other common trade name: *Inapetyl*
Indications: Adjunct to diet plan to reduce weight
Category: Anorexiant; CNS Stimulant; Sympathomimetic amine
Half-life: N/A
Clinically important, potentially hazardous interactions with: furazolidone, guanethidine, MAO inhibitors, SSRIs

Reactions

Skin
Allergic reactions (sic)
Diaphoresis
Erythema
Rash (sic)
Urticaria

Hair
Hair – alopecia

Cardiovascular
Flushing

Other
Anxiety
Depression (following withdrawal)
Dizziness
Gynecomastia
Headache
Hypersensitivity
Myalgia
Tremor
Xerostomia

BERGAMOT*

Scientific name: *Citrus aurantium ssp bergamia*
Family: Rutaceae
Trade and other common names: Bergamottin; Earl Grey tea; Florida Water; Kananga Water; Neroli oil; Oil of bergamot
Category: Mild stimulant
Purported indications and other uses: Headache, bronchitis, vitiligo, mycosis fungoides, psoriasis (in conjunction with UVA), insecticide, essential oil in perfumery, cosmetics, flavoring
Half-life: N/A

*Note: two distinct species are known by the common name of bergamot. This profile does not refer to *Monarda didyma*

Reactions

Skin
  Adverse effects (sic) [1]
  Berloque dermatitis [2]
  Bullous eruption [1]
  Burning [1]
  Dermatitis [2]

Erythema [1]
Photosensitivity [3]
Phototoxicity [7]
Pigmentation [1]
Tumors [1]
Vesiculation [1]

Note: Oil of bergamot possesses photosensitive and melanogenic properties because of the presence of furocoumarins, primarily bergapten (5-methoxypsoralen [5-MOP]). Its use is restricted or banned in many countries

BLACK COHOSH

Scientific names: *Actaea macrotys; Actaea racemosa; Cimicifuga racemosa*
Family: Ranunculaceae
Trade and other common names: Baneberry; Black Snake root; Bugbane; Bugwort; Macrotys; Rattletop; Rattleweed; Remifemin (PhytoPharmica/Enzymatic Therapy; Schaper & Brummer); Shengma; Squawroot
Category: Phytoestrogen
Purported indications and other uses: Anxiety, arthritis, asthma, cardiovascular and circulatory problems, climacteric, menstrual and premenstrual disorders, colds, cough, constipation, depression, kidney disorders, malaria, sore throat, tinnitus
Half-life: N/A
Clinically important, potentially hazardous interactions with: estrogens, salicylates, tamoxifen

Reactions

Skin
  Diaphoresis [2]

Jaundice [1]
Petechiae (forearms)

Pruritus [1]

Rash (sic) [1]

Other

Arthralgia (overdose)

Dizziness [1]

Mastodynia [1]

Seizures [3]

Tremor (overdose)

Note: In 2001, the American College of Obstetricians and Gynecologists stated that black cohosh might be helpful in the short term (6 months or less) for women with vasomotor symptoms of menopause

BLUE COHOSH

Scientific name: *Caulophyllum thalictroides*
Family: Berberidaceae
Trade and other common names: Beechdrops; Blue ginseng; Blueberry root; Papoose root; Squawroot; Yellow ginseng
Category: Anthelmintic; Antispasmodic diuretic; Diaphoretic; Expectorant; Oxytocic
Purported indications and other uses: Rheumatism, dropsy, epilepsy, hysteria, uterine inflammation, thrush, menopause, headache, sexual debility, aphthous stomatitis, laxative, colic, sore throat, hiccups
Half-life: N/A
Clinically important, potentially hazardous interactions with: cardioactive drugs

Reactions

Skin

Allergic reactions (sic)

Diaphoresis [1]

Other

Mucosal irritation

Myalgia [1]

Shock [1]

Note: Cohosh is from the Algonquin word 'rough', referring to the appearance of the roots. It is a toxic herb and should not be confused with the safer, unrelated herb, Black Cohosh

BUPROPION

Trade names: Wellbutrin (GSK); Zyban (GSK)
Indications: Depression, aid to smoking cessation
Category: Aid to smoking cessation; Heterocyclic antidepressant
Half-life: 14 hours
Clinically important, potentially hazardous interactions with: cyclosporine, isocarboxazid, phenelzine, ritonavir, tranylcypromine, trimipramine

Reactions

Skin

Acne (1–10%)

Angioedema

Diaphoresis (5%) [2]

Edema (>1%) [1]
Erythema multiforme [3]
Exanthems (<0.1%) [2]
Exfoliative dermatitis
Lupus panniculitis [1]
Peripheral edema [1]
Photosensitivity (<0.1%)
Pruritus (4%) [3]
Rash (sic) (4%) [2]
Stevens–Johnson syndrome
Urticaria [11]
Xerosis (1–10%)

Hair
Hair – alopecia (<1%) [1]
Hair – hirsutism (1–10%)
Hair – pigmentation (<1%)

Hematopoietic
Ecchymoses (<0.1%)

Cardiovascular
Chest pain [1]
Flushing (4%)
Hot flashes

Other
Anaphylactoid reactions [1]
Arthralgia [1]
Ballism [1]
Bromhidrosis

Bruxism (<0.1%)
Death [2]
Delusions [1]
DRESS syndrome [1]
Dysgeusia (4%) [1]
Gingivitis
Glossitis
Gynecomastia (<1%)
Hallucinations [1]
Headache
Hyperesthesia (<0.1%)
Hypersensitivity [5]
Myalgia (6%) [2]
Oral edema (<1%)
Paresthesias (2%)
Parkinsonism [1]
Priapism [1]
Psychosis [1]
Rhabdomyolysis [1]
Seizures [15]
Serum sickness [8]
Sialorrhea
Stomatitis (>1%)
Tinnitus
Tongue edema (0.1%) [1]
Tremor (>10%) [1]
Twitching (2%)
Vaginitis
Xerostomia (up to 64%) [12]

BUSPIRONE

Trade name: BuSpar (Bristol-Myers Squibb)
Other common trade names: *Ansail; Apo-Buspirone; Bespar; Biron; Busirone; Bustab; Kallmiren; Narol; Neurosine; Nu-Buspirone*
Indications: Anxiety
Category: Nonbenzodiazepine anxiolytic tranquilizer; Serotonin antagonist
Half-life: 2–3 hours
Clinically important, potentially hazardous interactions with: grapefruit juice, nefazodone, ritonavir, **St John's wort**

Reactions

Skin
Acne (<0.1%)

Bullous eruption (<1%)
Diaphoresis [1]

Edema
Exanthems
Facial edema (1%)
Hypomelanosis [1]
Photo-recall [1]
Pruritus (1%)
Pseudoparkinsonism [1]
Purpura (1%)
Rash (sic) (<1%)
Seborrheic dermatitis [1]
Urticaria (<1%)
Xerosis (1%)

Hair
Hair – alopecia (1%) [2]

Nails
Nails – thinning (<0.1%)

Hematopoietic
Ecchymoses

Cardiovascular
Congestive heart failure [1]
Flushing

Other
Dysgeusia (<1%)
Galactorrhea (<0.1%)
Glossodynia
Glossopyrosis
Headache
Myalgia
Paresthesias (1%) [1]
Parkinsonism [1]
Parosmia (1%)
Serotonin syndrome [2]
Sialorrhea
Sicca syndrome [1]
Tinnitus
Xerostomia (3%)

BUTABARBITAL

Trade names: Butalan; Buticaps; Butisol (MedPointe)
Other common trade name: *Day-Barb*
Indications: Sedation
Category: Sedative-hypnotic barbiturate
Half-life: 40–140 hours
Clinically important, potentially hazardous interactions with: alcohol, antihistamines, ardeparin, argatroban, brompheniramine, buclizine, chlorpheniramine, dalteparin, danaparoid, dicumarol, enoxaparin, ethanolamine, heparin, imatinib, tinzaparin, warfarin

Reactions

Skin
Acne
Angioedema (<1%)
Bullous eruption [1]
Erythema multiforme [1]
Exanthems [1]
Exfoliative dermatitis (<1%) [1]
Fixed eruption [1]
Herpes simplex
Lupus erythematosus [2]
Necrosis [1]
Photosensitivity [1]
Pruritus
Purpura [1]
Rash (sic) (<1%)
Stevens–Johnson syndrome (<1%)
Toxic epidermal necrolysis [1]
Urticaria
Vasculitis

Other
Oral ulceration
Porphyria variegata
Rhabdomyolysis [1]
Thrombophlebitis (<1%)

BUTALBITAL

Trade names: Esgic (Forest); Fioricet (Watson); Fiorinal (Watson)
Other common trade names: *Amaphen; Anoquan; Axotal; Butace; Fioricet; Marnal; Medigesic; Phrenilin; Tecnal*
Indications: Tension headaches
Category: Sedative-analgesic barbiturate
Half-life: 35 hours
Clinically important, potentially hazardous interactions with: alcohol, dicumarol

Reactions

Skin
  Bullous eruption [1]
  Erythema multiforme [2]
  Exanthems [1]
  Exfoliative dermatitis (<1%) [1]
  Fixed eruption [1]
  Herpes simplex
  Lupus erythematosus [2]
  Necrosis [1]
  Photosensitivity [1]
  Pruritus
  Purpura [1]
  Rash (sic) (1–10%)

  Stevens–Johnson syndrome (<1%)
  Toxic epidermal necrolysis [1]
  Urticaria [1]
  Vasculitis

Other
  Anaphylactoid reactions (1–10%)
  Headache
  Oral erythema multiforme [1]
  Oral ulceration
  Porphyria variegata
  Rhabdomyolysis [1]

BUTORPHANOL

Trade name: Stadol (Bristol-Myers Squibb)
Other common trade names: *Biforal; Busphen; Stadol NS*
Indications: Pain, migraine
Category: Analgesic; Narcotic
Half-life: 2.5–4 hours
Clinically important, potentially hazardous interactions with: cimetidine

Reactions

Skin
  Clammy skin
  Diaphoresis (1–10%)
  Edema (<1%)
  Exanthems
  Gooseflesh
  Pruritus (1–10%) [2]
  Rash (sic) (<1%)
  Urticaria (<1%)

Cardiovascular
  Flushing (1–10%)

Other
  Dysgeusia (3–9%)
  Headache
  Injection-site reactions (sic)
  Paresthesias
  Tinnitus
  Xerostomia (3–9%)

CARBAMAZEPINE

Trade names: Carbatrol; Epitol (Teva); Tegretol (Novartis)
Other common trade names: *Apo-Carbamazepine; Atreol; Foxsalepsin; Kodapan; Lexin; Mazepine; Sirtal; Tegretol XR; Teril; Timonil*
Indications: Epilepsy, pain or trigeminal neuralgia
Category: Anticonvulsant; Antimanic; Antineuralgic; Antipsychotic
Half-life: 18–55 hours
Clinically important, potentially hazardous interactions with: acetylcysteine, adenosine, aprepitant, aripiprazole, **caffeine**, charcoal, clarithromycin, clorazepate, clozapine, delavirdine, diltiazem, doxacurium, erythromycin, felodipine, fosamprenavir, imatinib, **influenza vaccines**, midazolam, solifenacin, **St John's wort**, telithromycin, troleandomycin, verapamil, voriconazole

Reactions

Skin
Acne keloid [1]
Acute generalized exanthematous pustulosis (AGEP) [5]
Adverse effects (sic) [1]
Allergic reactions (sic) [5]
Angioedema (<1%) [4]
Anticonvulsant hypersensitivity syndrome [8]
Bullous eruption (<1%) [4]
Collagen disease [1]
Dermatitis [7]
Diaphoresis (1–10%)
Eczema [2]
Edema
Eosinophilic pustular folliculitis (Ofuji's disease) [1]
Epidermolysis bullosa [1]
Erythema (sheet-like)
Erythema [1]
Erythema multiforme [17]
Erythema nodosum (<1%)
Erythroderma [12]
Exanthems (>5%) [25]
Exfoliative dermatitis [22]
Facial edema [1]
Fixed eruption (<1%) [9]
Lichenoid eruption [6]
Linear IgA dermatosis [1]
Lupus erythematosus [29]

Lymphoma [2]
Mucocutaneous lymph node syndrome (Kawasaki syndrome) [2]
Mycosis fungoides [3]
Pemphigus [1]
Peripheral edema [2]
Petechiae [1]
Photosensitivity [9]
Pigmentation
Pruritus (<1%) [6]
Pseudo-mycosis fungoides [1]
Psoriasis [1]
Purpura [8]
Pustules [5]
Rash (sic) (>10%) [14]
Schamberg's disease
Side effects (sic) [2]
Stevens–Johnson syndrome (1–10%) [32]
Toxic epidermal necrolysis (1–10%) [37]
Toxic pustuloderma (probably AGEP [ed]) [3]
Toxic-allergic shock [1]
Toxicoderma [1]
Urticaria [12]
Vasculitis [5]

Hair
Hair – alopecia [6]

Nails
Nails – discoloration (bluish-black) [1]

Nails – hypoplasia [1]
Nails – lichen planus [1]
Nails – loss [1]
Nails – onychomadesis [1]

Eyes
Dyschromatopsia [1]
Periorbital edema [1]

Cardiovascular
Bradycardia [3]
Coronary artery disorders [1]
Tachycardia [1]

Other
Acute intermittent porphyria [5]
Death [1]
DRESS syndrome [5]
Dysgeusia [1]
Fetal anticonvulsant syndrome [1]
Glossitis
Headache

Hypersensitivity [47]
Lymphoproliferative disease [5]
Mania [1]
Mucocutaneous eruption [4]
Oral lichenoid eruption [1]
Oral mucosal eruption [1]
Oral ulceration [2]
Porphyria cutanea tarda [1]
Porphyria variegata [1]
Pseudolymphoma [15]
Rhabdomyolysis [1]
Seizures [2]
Serum sickness [1]
Stomatitis
test
Thrombophlebitis
Tinnitus
Tongue ulceration [2]
Xerostomia

CHLORAL HYDRATE

Synonyms: chloral; hydrated chloral
Trade names: Aquachloral; Noctec
Other common trade names: *Chloraldurat; Medianox; Novochlorhydrate; Somnox; Welldorm*
Indications: Insomnia, sedation
Category: Sedative-hypnotic
Half-life: 8–11 hours
Clinically important, potentially hazardous interactions with: antihistamines, azatadine, azelastine, brompheniramine, buclizine, chlorpheniramine, clemastine, dexchlorpheniramine, diphenhydramine, meclizine, tripelennamine

Reactions

Skin
Acne [2]
Angioedema [2]
Bullous eruption [1]
Dermatitis [2]
Eczema [1]
Erythema [1]
Erythema multiforme [2]
Exanthems [3]
Fixed eruption [5]

Lichenoid eruption [1]
Perioral dermatitis [1]
Pruritus [2]
Purpura [2]
Rash (sic) (1–10%)
Ulcerations [1]
Urticaria (1–10%) [2]

Cardiovascular
Flushing [1]

QT prolongation [1]

Other

Acute intermittent porphyria

Death [2]

Dysgeusia

Headache

Hypersensitivity

Oral lesions [2]

Oral ulceration [1]

Stomatitis [1]

CHLORDIAZEPOXIDE

Trade names: Libritabs (Valeant); Librium (Valeant); Limbitrol (Valeant)

Other common trade names: *Corax; Huberplex; Medilium; Mitran; Multum; Novopoxide; Psicofar; Reposans-10; Solium; Tropium*

Indications: Anxiety

Category: Antianxiety; Antipanic; Antitremor ; Benzodiazepine sedative-hypnotic

Half-life: 6–25 hours

Clinically important, potentially hazardous interactions with: chlorpheniramine, clarithromycin, efavirenz, esomeprazole, imatinib, indinavir, ketoconazole, nelfinavir, ritonavir

Limbitrol is amitriptyline and chlordiazepoxide

Reactions

Skin

Angioedema (<1%) [2]

Dermatitis (1–10%)

Diaphoresis (>10%)

Edema (1–10%)

Erythema multiforme (<1%) [5]

Erythema nodosum (<1%) [2]

Exanthems [2]

Fixed eruption (<1%) [6]

Lupus erythematosus [3]

Photosensitivity [6]

Pigmented purpuric eruption [1]

Pruritus [1]

Purpura [5]

Rash (sic) (>10%) [1]

Urticaria [4]

Vasculitis [2]

Hair

Hair – alopecia [3]

Other

Acute intermittent porphyria [1]

Galactorrhea [3]

Gynecomastia [1]

Headache

Injection-site phlebitis

Paresthesias

Porphyria [1]

Sialopenia (>10%)

Sialorrhea (1–10%)

Xerostomia (>10%)

CHLORMEZANONE

Trade name: Trancopal
Indications: Anxiety
Category: Antianxiety
Half-life: 24 hours

Reactions

Skin
Edema
Erythema multiforme
Exanthems [2]
Fixed eruption [13]
Peripheral edema
Pruritus [1]
Rash (sic) [1]
Stevens–Johnson syndrome [2]
Toxic epidermal necrolysis [8]

Urticaria

Cardiovascular
Flushing

Other
Acute intermittent porphyria
Death
Dysgeusia [1]
Xerostomia [1]

CHLORPROMAZINE

Trade name: Thorazine (GSK)
Other common trade names: *Chloractil; Chlorazin; Chlorpromanyl; Esmino; Largactil; Novo-Chlorpromazine; Ormazine; Propaphenin; Prozin*
Indications: Psychosis, manic-depressive disorders
Category: Phenothiazine antipsychotic
Half-life: initial: 2 hours; terminal: 30 hours
Clinically important, potentially hazardous interactions with: alcohol, antihistamines, arsenic, chlorpheniramine, dofetilide, epinephrine, **evening primrose**, guanethidine, quinolones, sparfloxacin

Note: The prolonged use of chlorpromazine can produce a gray-blue or purplish pigmentation over light-exposed areas. This is a result of either dermal deposits of melanin, a chlorpromazine metabolite, or to a combination of both. Chlorpromazine melanosis is seen more often in women

Reactions

Skin
Angioedema (<1%) [1]
Bullous eruption (<1%) [1]
Dermatitis [1]
Erythema multiforme (<1%) [1]
Exanthems (>5%) [8]
Exfoliative dermatitis [1]
Fixed eruption (<1%)

Hypohidrosis (>10%)
Lichenoid eruption [1]
Lupus erythematosus [11]
Miliaria [1]
Peripheral edema
Photosensitivity (1–10%) [22]
Phototoxicity [6]
Pigmentation (<1%) [14]

Pruritus (1–10%) [2]
Purpura [6]
Pustules [1]
Rash (sic) (1–10%)
Seborrheic dermatitis [4]
Toxic epidermal necrolysis (<1%) [2]
Urticaria [5]
Vasculitis [3]
Xerosis

Nails

Nails – photo-onycholysis [1]
Nails – pigmentation [4]

Eyes

Cataract [1]
Corneal opacity [1]

Cardiovascular

Hypotension [1]
QT prolongation [1]

Tachycardia [1]

Other

Anaphylactoid reactions (<1%) [1]
Death [1]
Galactorrhea (1–10%)
Gynecomastia (1–10%)
Headache
Injection-site aseptic necrosis
Mastodynia (1–10%)
Oral mucosal eruption
Oral pigmentation
Oral ulceration
Polyarteritis nodosa [1]
Priapism (<1%) [2]
Pseudolymphoma [1]
Tremor [1]
Xerostomia (1–10%)

CITALOPRAM

Synonym: nitalapram
Trade name: Celexa (Forest)
Indications: Depression, obsessive-compulsive disorder, panic disorder
Category: Selective serotonin reuptake inhibitor (SSRI)
Half-life: 33 hours
Clinically important, potentially hazardous interactions with: isocarboxazid, MAO
inhibitors, phenelzine, selegiline, **St John's wort**, sumatriptan, tramadol, tranylcypromine,
trazodone

Reactions

Skin

Cellulitis
Dermatitis
Diaphoresis (11%) [2]
Eczema
Exanthems [1]
Facial edema
Hypohidrosis
Neuroleptic malignant syndrome [1]
Photosensitivity
Pigmentation [1]

Pruritus (<10%) [1]
Pruritus ani et vulvae
Psoriasis [1]
Purpura [1]
Rash (sic) (<10%)
Urticaria
Vasculitis [1]
Xerosis

Hair

Hair – alopecia
Hair – hypertrichosis

Eyes
  Ocular side effects (sic) [1]

Cardiovascular
  Bradycardia [1]
  Hot flashes
  Hypotension [1]
  QT prolongation [1]
  Torsades de pointes [1]

Other
  Anxiety [1]
  Bruxism [1]
  Death [4]
  Dizziness [1]
  Dysgeusia
  Galactorrhea [1]

  Gingivitis
  Gynecomastia
  Headache [1]
  Hyperesthesia
  Mastodynia
  Myalgia (>2%)
  Paresthesias
  Parkinsonism [1]
  Priapism (clitoral) [4]
  Serotonin syndrome [6]
  Sialorrhea [1]
  Stomatitis
  Tremor (jaw) [1]
  Twitching [1]
  Xerostomia (20%) [2]

CLOMIPRAMINE

Trade name: Anafranil (Mallinckrodt)
Other common trade names: *Anafranil Retard; Apo-Clomipramine; Clofranil; Clopress; Placil*
Indications: Obsessive-compulsive disorder
Category: Tricyclic antidepressant
Half-life: 21–31 hours
Clinically important, potentially hazardous interactions with: amprenavir, arbutamine, clonidine, epinephrine, formoterol, guanethidine, isocarboxazid, linezolid, MAO inhibitors, phenelzine, quinolones, sparfloxacin, tranylcypromine

Reactions

Skin
  Acne (2%)
  Allergic reactions (sic) (<3%)
  Cellulitis (2%)
  Cheilitis
  Chloasma
  Dermatitis (2%) [1]
  Diaphoresis (29%) [2]
  Edema (2%)
  Erythema
  Exanthems
  Folliculitis
  Photosensitivity (<1%) [3]
  Pigmentation (pseudocyanotic) [1]

  Pruritus (6%)
  Psoriasis
  Purpura (3%)
  Pustules
  Rash (sic) (8%)
  Seborrhea
  Urticaria (1%)
  Vasculitis
  Xerosis (2%)

Hair
  Hair – alopecia (<1%)
  Hair – alopecia areata [1]
  Hair – hypertrichosis

Cardiovascular
  Bradycardia [1]
  Flushing (8%)
  QT prolongation [1]

Other
  Ageusia
  Black tongue
  Dysgeusia (8%)
  Galactorrhea (<1%)
  Gingivitis
  Glossitis

Gynecomastia (2%)
Headache
Mastodynia (1%)
Myalgia (13%)
Paresthesias
Sialorrhea
Stomatitis
Tongue ulceration
Vaginitis (2%)
Xerostomia (84%) [4]

CLONAZEPAM

Trade name: Klonopin (Roche)
Other common trade names: *Clonex; Iktorivil; Landsen; Lonazep; Rivotril*
Indications: Petit mal and myoclonic seizures
Category: Benzodiazepine anticonvulsant
Half-life: 18–50 hours
Clinically important, potentially hazardous interactions with: amprenavir, chlorpheniramine, clarithromycin, efavirenz, esomeprazole, imatinib, indinavir, nelfinavir, oxycodone

Reactions

Skin
  Allergic reactions (sic) (1–10%)
  Angioedema [1]
  Dermatitis (1–10%)
  Diaphoresis (>10%)
  Erythema multiforme [1]
  Exanthems [1]
  Facial edema
  Hypermelanosis [1]
  Peripheral edema
  Pruritus
  Pseudo-mycosis fungoides [1]
  Purpura [1]
  Rash (sic) (>10%)
  Urticaria

Hair
  Hair – alopecia [1]

Hair – hirsutism

Other
  Black tongue [1]
  Burning mouth syndrome [1]
  Death [1]
  Dysgeusia [1]
  Gingivitis
  Headache
  Injection-site phlebitis
  Injection-site thrombosis
  Oral mucosal eruption [1]
  Oral ulceration
  Paresthesias
  Pseudolymphoma [2]
  Sialopenia (>10%)
  Sialorrhea (1–10%)
  Xerostomia (>10%) [1]

CLORAZEPATE

Trade name: Tranxene (Ovation) (Abbott)
Other common trade names: *Gen-XENE; Novoclopate; Transene; Tranxal; Tranxen; Tranxilen; Tranxilium*
Indications: Anxiety and panic disorders
Category: Anxiolytic ; Benzodiazepine sedative-hypnotic
Half-life: 48–96 hours
Clinically important, potentially hazardous interactions with: amprenavir, antacids, carbamazepine, carmustine, chlorpheniramine, clarithromycin, efavirenz, esomeprazole, imatinib, indinavir, itraconazole, ketoconazole, MAO inhibitors, midazolam, moclobemide, nelfinavir, phenytoin, sucralfate, theophylline, warfarin

Reactions

Skin
  Dermatitis (1–10%)
  Diaphoresis (>10%)
  Exanthems [1]
  Photosensitivity [1]
  Pruritus
  Purpura
  Rash (sic) (>10%)
  Urticaria [1]
  Vasculitis [1]
  Vesiculation [1]

Nails
  Nails – photo-onycholysis [1]

Other
  Headache
  Oral ulceration
  Paresthesias
  Porphyria [1]
  Sialopenia (>10%)
  Sialorrhea (1–10%)
  Tremor
  Xerostomia (>10%)

CLOZAPINE

Trade name: Clozaril (Novartis)
Other common trade names: *Entumin; Entumine; Leponex; Lozapin; Sizopin*
Indications: Schizophrenia
Category: Tricyclic antipsychotic
Half-life: 8–12 hours
Clinically important, potentially hazardous interactions with: **caffeine**, carbamazepine, fluoxetine, **guarana**, risperidone, ritonavir, selenium

Reactions

Skin
  Acute febrile neutrophilic dermatosis
    (Sweet's syndrome) [1]
  Acute generalized exanthematous
    pustulosis (AGEP) [1]

Allergic reactions (sic) [1]
Dermatitis (<1%)
Diaphoresis (6%) [4]
Eczema (<1%) [1]
Edema (<1%)

Erythema (<1%)
Erythema multiforme (<1%)
Exanthems [1]
Facial erosions [1]
Lupus erythematosus [1]
Neuroleptic malignant syndrome [4]
Nodular eruption [1]
Petechiae (<1%) [1]
Photosensitivity [1]
Pruritus (<1%)
Purpura (<1%)
Rash (sic) (2%)
Stevens–Johnson syndrome (<1%)
Urticaria (<1%)
Vasculitis (<1%)

Eyes
Periorbital edema (<1%)

Cardiovascular
Atrial fibrillation [1]
Congestive heart failure [1]

Other
Death [5]
Diabetes mellitus [1]
Dysgeusia (<1%)
Fever [1]
Glossodynia (1%)
Headache
Mastodynia (<1%)
Priapism [4]
Rhabdomyolysis [2]
Seizures [4]
Sialorrhea (31%) [19]
Tardive dyskinesia [1]
Tremor (1–10%) [1]
Xerostomia (6%) [3]

COCAINE

Trade name: Cocaine
Indications: Topical anesthesia
Category: Substance abuse drug; Topical anesthetic
Half-life: 75 minutes
Clinically important, potentially hazardous interactions with: epinephrine

Note: Cocaine is a benzoylmethylecogonine alkaloid derived from the leaves of the *Erythroxylon coca* tree. Street names for cocaine include: coke; flake; snow; toot, etc. Crack cocaine is a highly potent smokable form of cocaine

Reactions

Skin
Angioedema [2]
Bullous eruption [1]
Diaphoresis
Formication
Granulomas (foreign body) [1]
Hyperkeratosis (fingers and palms) [1]
Necrosis [3]
Nodular eruption [1]
Scleroderma (reversible) [3]
Stevens–Johnson syndrome [1]

Urticaria [1]
Vasculitis [1]
Warts (snorters' warts) [1]

Cardiovascular
Angina [2]
Chest pain [2]
Coronary artery disorders [6]

Other
Ageusia (>10%)
Anosmia (>10%)

Black tongue [1]

Bruxism [1]

Gingival ulceration [1]

Injection-site scarring [1]

Nasal septal perforation [3]

Necrosis of palate [1]

Porphyria [1]

Priapism [2]

Rhabdomyolysis [11]

Thrombophlebitis [1]

Tremor (1–10%)

COMFREY

Scientific names: *Symphytum asperum; Symphytum officinale; Symphytum x uplandicum; Symphytum. peregrinum*

Family: Boraginaceae

Trade and other common names: Ass ear; Blackwort; Boneset ; Bruisewort; consolida; consormol; consound; gum plant; knitback; Knitback; Knitbone; nipbone; Russian comfrey; Slippery Root; Wallwort

Category: Carminative

Purported indications and other uses: Leaf: Gastric and duodenal ulcer, rheumatic pain, gout, arthritis. Topical: poultice for bruises, sprains, athlete's foot, crural ulcers, mastitis, varicose ulcers. **Root**: Gastric and duodenal ulcers, hematemesis, colitis, diarrhea. Topical: ulcers, wounds, fractures, hernia

Half-life: N/A

Clinically important, potentially hazardous interactions with: eucalyptus

Reactions

Other

Budd–Chiari syndrome [3]

Death [2]

Toxicity [1]

Tumors [1]

Note: The FDA warns that comfrey contains pyrrolizidine alkaloids that can cause cirrhosis and liver failure when taken orally in high doses. It is banned in Germany and Canada. Topical application is safer and more effective; allantoin in comfrey stimulates cell proliferation, accelerating wound healing

DESIPRAMINE

Other common trade names: *Deprexan; Nebril; Nortimil; Pertofran; Pertofrane; Petylyl; PMS-Desipramine*
Indications: Depression
Category: Tricyclic antidepressant
Half-life: 7–60 hours
Clinically important, potentially hazardous interactions with: amprenavir, arbutamine, clonidine, epinephrine, fluoxetine, formoterol, guanethidine, isocarboxazid, linezolid, MAO inhibitors, phenelzine, quinolones, sparfloxacin, tranylcypromine

Reactions

Skin
  Acne
  Allergic reactions (sic) (<1%) [2]
  Angioedema [1]
  Diaphoresis (1–10%) [1]
  Edema
  Erythema
  Exanthems [5]
  Exfoliative dermatitis [1]
  Petechiae [1]
  Photosensitivity (1.4%) [1]
  Pigmentation (blue-gray) (photosensitive)
    [2]
  Pruritus [4]
  Purpura [2]
  Rash (sic) [1]
  Side effects (sic) [1]
  Urticaria [3]
  Vasculitis
  Xerosis

Hair
  Hair – alopecia (<1%) [1]

Hematopoietic
  Ecchymoses [1]

Cardiovascular
  Flushing [1]

Other
  Black tongue
  Bromhidrosis
  Dysgeusia (>10%)
  Galactorrhea (<1%)
  Gynecomastia (<1%)
  Hypersensitivity
  Mucous membrane desquamation [1]
  Paresthesias
  Pseudolymphoma [2]
  Stomatitis
  Tinnitus
  Xerostomia (>10%) [3]

DEXMEDETOMIDINE

Trade name: Precedex (Abbott)
Indications: Sedation for intensive care unit intubation
Category: Alpha-adrenoceptor blocker; Sedative
Half-life: 2 hours

Reactions

Skin
  Diaphoresis (<1%)
  Infections (2%)
  Xerosis

Eyes
  Photopsia (<1%)

Other
  Pain (3%)
  Sialopenia [1]

DEXTROAMPHETAMINE

Trade names: Adderall (Shire); Dexedrine (Alliant)
Other common trade names: *Dexamphetamine; Dexamphetamini; Dextrostat; Ferndex; Oxydess*
Indications: Narcolepsy, attention deficit disorder (ADD)
Category: Amphetamine; Central nervous system stimulant
Half-life: 10–12 hours
Clinically important, potentially hazardous interactions with: fluoxetine, fluvoxamine, MAO inhibitors, paroxetine, phenelzine, sertraline, tranylcypromine

Reactions

Skin
  Chills
  Diaphoresis (1–10%)
  Rash (sic) (<1%)
  Toxic epidermal necrolysis [1]
  Urticaria (<1%)

Other
  Dysgeusia
  Headache
  Rhabdomyolysis [10]
  Xerostomia (1–10%)

DIAZEPAM

Trade names: Diastat (Xcel); Dizac; Valium (Roche)
Other common trade names: *Assival; Dialar; Diapax; Diazemuls; Ducene; E-Pam; Meval; Novazam; Solis; Vivol*
Indications: Anxiety
Category: Anxiolytic; Benzodiazepine sedative-hypnotic
Half-life: 20–70 hours
Clinically important, potentially hazardous interactions with: alcohol, amprenavir, barbiturates, chlorpheniramine, clarithromycin, CNS depressants, efavirenz, esomeprazole, **eucalyptus**, fluoroquinolones, imatinib, indinavir, ivermectin, macrolide antibiotics, MAO inhibitors, methadone, nalbuphine, narcotics, nelfinavir, phenothiazines, ritonavir, SSRIs

Reactions

Skin

Acne [1]
Allergic reactions (sic) [2]
Angioedema [1]
Bullous eruption [1]
Dermatitis (1–10%) [3]
Diaphoresis (>10%)
Eczema [1]
Exanthems [6]
Exfoliative dermatitis [2]
Fixed eruption (<1%) [2]
Granuloma disciformis (Miescher) [1]
Melanoma [1]
Peripheral edema [1]
Pigmentation [2]
Pruritus [1]
Purpura [4]
Rash (sic) (>10%) [1]
Urticaria [1]
Vasculitis [1]

Nails

Nails – parrot-beak [1]

Cardiovascular

Flushing [1]
Hypotension [1]

Other

Anaphylactoid reactions [1]
Dizziness [1]
Gynecomastia [3]
Headache
Hypersensitivity [1]
Injection-site pain [1]
Injection-site phlebitis (>10%) [2]
Paresthesias
Porphyria [2]
Porphyria variegata
Rhabdomyolysis [1]
Sialorrhea
Tongue furry
Xerostomia (>10%)

DIETHYLPROPION

Synonym: amfepramone
Trade name: Tenuate (Sanofi-Aventis)
Other common trade names: *Anorex; Linea; Nobesine; Prefamone; Regenon; Tenuate Retard; Tepanil*
Indications: Weight reduction
Category: Anorexiant; CNS stimulant
Half-life: 4–6 hours
Clinically important, potentially hazardous interactions with: fluoxetine, fluvoxamine, MAO inhibitors, paroxetine, phenelzine, sertraline, tranylcypromine

Reactions

Skin
  Diaphoresis (<1%)
  Erythema (<1%)
  Erythema multiforme [1]
  Exanthems (<1%)
  Pruritus (<1%)
  Purpura (<1%)
  Rash (sic)
  Scleroderma [2]
  Systemic sclerosis [1]
  Urticaria

Hair
  Hair – alopecia (<1%)

Hematopoietic
  Ecchymoses

Cardiovascular
  Flushing (<1%)

Other
  Dysgeusia
  Gynecomastia
  Headache
  Myalgia (<1%)
  Tremor
  Xerostomia

DIPHENHYDRAMINE

Trade names: Allermax; Benadryl (Pfizer); Benylin; Compoz; Sominex 2; Valdrene
Other common trade names: *Allerdryl; Allermin; Banophen; Benahist; Dibrondrin; Dolestan; Genahist; Insomnal; Nytol; Resmin; Sediat*
Indications: Allergic rhinitis, urticaria
Category: Antidyskinetic; Antiemetic; Antihistamine; Sedative-hypnotic
Half-life: 2–8 hours
Clinically important, potentially hazardous interactions with: alcohol, anticholinergics, chloral hydrate, CNS depressants, glutethimide, MAO inhibitors

Reactions

Skin
  Allergic reactions (sic) [1]
  Angioedema (<1%) [1]
  Dermatitis [4]

Diaphoresis
Eczema [2]
Edema (<1%)
Exanthems [1]

Fixed eruption [4]
Livedo reticularis [1]
Photosensitivity (<1%) [4]
Pruritus [3]
Purpura [1]
Rash (sic) (<1%)
Toxic epidermal necrolysis [3]
Urticaria
Vasculitis [1]

Other
Anaphylactoid reactions [4]

Death [1]
Hypersensitivity
Injection-site gangrene [1]
Injection-site necrosis [1]
Myalgia (<1%)
Paresthesias (<1%)
Rhabdomyolysis [3]
Tinnitus
Tremor
Xerostomia (1–10%)

DISULFIRAM

Trade name: Antabuse (Odyssey)
Other common trade names: *Antabus; Busetal; Esperal; Nocbin; Refusal; Tetradin*
Indications: Alcoholism
Category: Deterrent to alcohol consumption
Half-life: N/A
Clinically important, potentially hazardous interactions with: alcohol, anisindione, anticoagulants, **capsicum**, cyclosporine, dicumarol, ethanolamine, ethotoin, fosphenytoin, mephenytoin, metronidazole, phenytoin, warfarin

Reactions

Skin
Acne [3]
Adverse effects (sic) (from beer-containing shampoo) [1]
Allergic reactions (sic)
Bullous eruption [2]
Dermatitis [16]
Diaphoresis (<1%) (with alcohol)
Eczema [2]
Exanthems [2]
Fixed eruption (<1%) [3]
Purpura [1]
Pustules [1]
Rash (sic) (1–10%)
Recall reaction (nickel) [4]

Toxic epidermal necrolysis [1]
Urticaria [3]
Vasculitis [1]
Yellow palms [1]

Cardiovascular
Atrial fibrillation [1]
Flushing (<1%) (with alcohol) [4]

Other
Dysgeusia (metallic or garlic aftertaste) (1–10%)
Headache
Hypogeusia
Paresthesias
Periarteritis nodosa [2]

DIVALPROEX (See VALPROIC ACID)

DONEPEZIL

Synonym: E2020
Trade name: Aricept (Eisai) (Endo)
Indications: Mild dementia of the Alzheimer's type
Category: Cholinergic ; Reversible acetylcholinesterase inhibitor for Alzheimer's disease
Half-life: 50–70 hours
Clinically important, potentially hazardous interactions with: galantamine

Reactions

Skin
  Dermatitis (<1%)
  Diaphoresis (>1%)
  Erythema (<1%)
  Facial edema (<1%)
  Hyperkeratosis (<1%)
  Neurodermatitis (<1%)
  Neuroleptic malignant syndrome [1]
  Pigmentation (<1%)
  Pruritus (>1%)
  Purpura (1–10%) [1]
  Striae (<1%)
  Ulcerations (<1%)
  Urticaria (>1%)

Hair
  Hair – alopecia (<1%)
  Hair – hirsutism (<1%)

Eyes
  Periorbital edema (<1%)

Hematopoietic
  Ecchymoses (4%)

Cardiovascular
  Atrial fibrillation [1]
  Flushing [1]

Other
  Anxiety [1]
  Depression [1]
  Dizziness [1]
  Dysgeusia (<1%)
  Fatigue [1]
  Gingivitis (<1%)
  Headache [1]
  Paresthesias (<1%)
  Rhinitis [1]
  Tongue edema (<1%)
  Vaginitis (<1%)
  Xerostomia (<1%)

DOXAPRAM

Trade name: Dopram (Baxter)
Indications: Chronic obstructive pulmonary disease, drug-induced CNS depression
Category: CNS stimulant; Respiratory stimulant
Duration of action: 3.4 hours

Reactions

Skin
  Diaphoresis (<1%)
  Pruritus [1]

Cardiovascular
  Flushing [1]

Other
  Injection-site erythema

Injection-site pain
Injection-site phlebitis (<1%)

Oral lesions
Paresthesias

DOXEPIN

Trade names: Sinequan (Pfizer); Zonalon (topical) (Bioglan)
Other common trade names: *Adapin; Alti-Doxepin; Anten; Aponal; Doneurin; Gilex; Mareen; Novo-Doxepin; Sinquan; Triadapin*
Indications: Mental depression, anxiety
Category: Antipanic; Tricyclic antidepressant
Half-life: 6–8 hours
Clinically important, potentially hazardous interactions with: alcohol, amprenavir, arbutamine, cholestyramine, clonidine, CNS depressants, epinephrine, formoterol, guanethidine, isocarboxazid, linezolid, MAO inhibitors, phenelzine, QT interval prolonging agents, quinolones, selegiline, sparfloxacin, sympathomimetics, tranylcypromine

Reactions

Skin

Allergic reactions (sic)
Dermatitis (from topical) [14]
Diaphoresis (1–10%)
Edema
Erythema
Erythroderma [1]
Exanthems [1]
Peripheral edema [1]
Photosensitivity (<1%) [2]
Pruritus [1]
Purpura [1]
Rash (sic) [1]
Toxic dermatitis [1]
Urticaria
Vasculitis

Hair

Hair – alopecia (<1%)

Cardiovascular

Flushing [1]

QT prolongation [1]

Other

Aphthous stomatitis [1]
Application-site burning
Application-site edema
Dysgeusia (>10%)
Galactorrhea (<1%)
Glossitis [1]
Glossodynia [1]
Gynecomastia (<1%)
Headache
Paresthesias
Parkinsonism
Pseudolymphoma [2]
Rhabdomyolysis [1]
Stomatitis [1]
Tinnitus
Tremor
Xerostomia (>10%) [3]

DROPERIDOL

Trade names: Droperidol; Inapsine (Akorn)
Other common trade names: *Dehydrobenzperidol; Droleptan; Inapsin; Sintodian*
Indications: Tranquilizer and antiemetic in surgical procedures
Category: Antiemetic; Antipsychotic
Half-life: 2.3 hours

Reactions

Skin
Chills
Diaphoresis
Pruritus [1]
Shivering

Cardiovascular
QT prolongation [1]

Other
Anxiety [1]
Death [3]
Seizures [1]

DULOXETINE

Trade name: Cymbalta (Lilly)
Indications: Depression
Category: Antidepressant; SSRI
Half-life: 8–17 hours
Clinically important, potentially hazardous interactions with: cimetidine, ciprofloxacin, enoxacin, fluoxetine, fluvoxamine, MAO inhibitors, paroxetine, quinidine, thioridazine

Reactions

Skin
Acne (<1%)
Diaphoresis (6%)
Eczema (<1%)
Erythema (<1%)
Facial edema (<1%)
Peripheral edema (<1%)
Photosensitivity (<1%)
Pruritus (<1%)
Purpura (<1%)
Rash (sic) (<1%)

Hair
Hair – alopecia (<1%)

Hematopoietic
Ecchymoses (<1%)

Cardiovascular
Hot flashes (2%)

Other
Abdominal pain (>2%)
Anxiety (3%)
Arthralgia (>2%)
Asthenia [1]
Back pain (>2%)
Cough (>2%)
Dizziness (9%) [3]
Dysphagia (<1%)
Fatigue [1]
Gingivitis (<1%)
Headache (>2%)
Pharyngitis (>2%)
Phlebitis (<1%)

Tremor (3%)   Xerostomia (15%) [2]
Upper respiratory infection (>2%)

EPHEDRA

Scientific names: *Ephedra equisetina; Ephedra intermedia; Ephedra sinica; Ephedra vulgaris*
Family: Gnetaceae
Trade and other common names: Joint Fir; Ma Huang; Popotillo; Sea Grape; Teamster's Tea;
Yellow Astringent; Yellow Horse
Category: Cardiovascular stimulant; CNS stimulant
Purported indications and other uses: Bronchospasm, asthma, bronchitis, allergy, appetite
suppressant, colds, flu, fever, chills, edema, headache, anhidrosis, diuretic, joint and bone pain
Half-life: N/A
Clinically important, potentially hazardous interactions with: acetazolamide, amitriptyline,
caffeine, corticosteriods, ephedrine, epinephrine, guanethidine, **guarana**, MAO inhibitors,
olmesartan, phenelzine, phenylpropanolamine, selegiline, sibutramine, sodium bicarbonate

Reactions

Skin   Eosinophilia–myalgia syndrome [1]
  Adverse effects (sic) [3]   Hypersensitivity
                                                               Seizures [4]
Cardiovascular   Side effects (sic) [1]
  Flushing   Tremor
                                                               Xerostomia [1]
Other
  Death [3]

Note: The FDA has recently banned Ephedra because of serious side effects

ESCITALOPRAM

Synonyms: Lu-26-054; S-Citalopram
Trade name: Lexapro (Forest)
Indications: Major depressive disorders, anxiety
Category: Antidepressant; Selective serotonin reuptake inhibitor (SSRI)
Half-life: 27–32 hours
Clinically important, potentially hazardous interactions with: alcohol, **kava**, MAO
inhibitors, selegiline, **St John's wort**, sumatriptan, **valerian**

Reactions

Skin   Diaphoresis (5%)
  Acne (<1%)   Eczema (<1%)
  Allergic reactions (sic) (1–10%)   Edema (<1%)
  Chills (<1%)   Facial edema
  Dermatitis   Flu-like syndrome (5%)

Folliculitis (<1%)
Furunculosis (<1%)
Peripheral edema
Pruritus (<1%)
Purpura (<1%)
Rash (sic) (1–10%)
Shivering
Xerosis (<1%)

Hair
Hair – alopecia (<1%)

Eyes
Conjunctivitis (<1%)

Cardiovascular
Flushing (<1%)
Hot flashes (1–10%)

Other
Anaphylactoid reactions
Anxiety (<1%)

Arthralgia (<1%)
Bruxism (<1%)
Cough (1–10%)
Depression (<1%)
Dizziness (5%)
Dysgeusia (<1%)
Headache
Limb pain (<1%)
Lipomatosis
Myalgia (1–10%)
Oral vesiculation (1–19%)
Paresthesias (1–10%)
Restless legs syndrome (<1%)
Tic disorder (<1%)
Tinnitus (1–10%)
Toothache (1–10%)
Tremor (1–10%)
Twitching (<1%)
Xerostomia (6%)

ESTAZOLAM

Trade name: ProSom
Other common trade names: *Domnamid; Esilgan; Eurodin; Kainever; Nuctalon; Tasedan*
Indications: Insomnia
Category: Benzodiazepine sedative-hypnotic
Half-life: 10–24 hours
Clinically important, potentially hazardous interactions with: indinavir, ritonavir

Reactions

Skin
Acne (<1%)
Allergic reactions (sic) (<1%)
Chills (<1%)
Dermatitis (<1%)
Diaphoresis (1–10%)
Edema (<1%)
Photosensitivity
Pruritus (1–10%)
Purpura (<1%)
Rash (sic) (>10%)
Urticaria (1–10%)
Xerosis (<1%)

Eyes
Eyelid edema (<1%)

Cardiovascular
Flushing (1–10%)

Other
Dysgeusia (1–10%)
Glossitis
Gynecomastia (<1%)
Myalgia (1–10%)
Oral ulceration (<1%)
Paresthesias (1–10%)
Sialopenia (>10%)

Sialorrhea (<1%)   Xerostomia (>10%)
Vaginal pruritus (1–10%)

ETHCHLORVYNOL

Other common trade names: *Arvynol; Nostel*
Indications: Insomnia
Category: Sedative-hypnotic
Half-life: 10–20 hours
Clinically important, potentially hazardous interactions with: antihistamines,
brompheniramine, buclizine, chlorpheniramine, clemastine, dexchlorpheniramine, meclizine,
tripelennamine

Reactions

Skin
  Allergic reactions (sic)
  Bullous eruption (from overdose) [2]
  Diaphoresis
  Fixed eruption [1]
  Pruritus
  Purpura [1]
  Rash (sic) (1–10%)
  Urticaria

Other
  Acute intermittent porphyria
  Death
  Dysgeusia (>10%)
  Facial numbness
  Hypersensitivity
  Paresthesias
  Pressure necrosis [1]

ETHOSUXIMIDE

Trade name: Zarontin (Pfizer)
Other common trade names: *Emeside; Ethymal; Petnidan; Pyknolepsinum; Simatin; Zarondan*
Indications: Absence (petit mal) seizures
Category: Succinimide anticonvulsant
Half-life: 50–60 hours

Reactions

Skin
  Anticonvulsant hypersensitivity syndrome
   [1]
  Erythema multiforme (<1%) [1]
  Exanthems (1–5%) [2]
  Exfoliative dermatitis (<1%)
  Lupus erythematosus (>10%) [19]
  Pruritus
  Purpura [1]

  Rash (sic) (<1%)
  Raynaud's phenomenon [3]
  Side effects (sic) (3.4%) [1]
  Stevens–Johnson syndrome (>10%) [1]
  Urticaria (1–5%) [1]

Hair
  Hair – alopecia
  Hair – hirsutism

Eyes
  Periorbital edema

Other
  Acute intermittent porphyria

Gingival hypertrophy
Headache
Oral ulceration
Tongue edema

ETHOTOIN

Trade name: Peganone (Ovation)
Other common trade name: *Accenon*
Indications: Tonic–clonic (grand mal) seizures
Category: Hydantoin anticonvulsant
Half-life: 3–9 hours
Clinically important, potentially hazardous interactions with: chloramphenicol, cyclosporine, disulfiram, dopamine, imatinib, itraconazole

Reactions

Skin
  Bullous eruption
  Fixed eruption
  Lupus erythematosus
  Purpura [1]

Rash (sic)

Other
  Gingival hypertrophy
  Pseudolymphoma [1]

FELBAMATE

Trade name: Felbatol (MedPointe)
Other common trade names: *Felbamyl; Taloxa*
Indications: Partial seizures
Category: Antiepileptic
Half-life: 13–23 hours

Reactions

Skin
  Acne (3.4%)
  Anticonvulsant hypersensitivity syndrome
    [1]
  Bullous eruption (<1%)
  Diaphoresis
  Edema
  Facial edema (3.4%)
  Idiosyncratic drug reactions [1]
  Lichen planus
  Livedo reticularis

Lupus erythematosus
Photosensitivity (<0.01%)
Pruritus (>1%)
Purpura
Pustules [1]
Rash (sic) (3.5%)
Stevens–Johnson syndrome [1]
Toxic epidermal necrolysis [1]
Urticaria (<1%)

Hair
  Hair – alopecia

Cardiovascular
 Flushing
 QT prolongation [1]

Other
 Anaphylactoid reactions (<0.01%)
 Dysgeusia (6.1%)
 Foetor ex ore (halitosis)

 Gingivitis
 Glossitis
 Headache
 Myalgia (2.6%)
 Oral edema (>1%)
 Paresthesias (3.5%)
 Thrombophlebitis
 Xerostomia (2.6%)

FENTANYL

Trade names: Actiq (Cephalon); Duragesic (Janssen)
Other common trade names: *Beatryl; Durogesic; Fentanest; Leptanal; Sublimaze*
Indications: Chronic pain
Category: Narcotic agonist analgesic
Half-life: 1.5–6 hours
Clinically important, potentially hazardous interactions with: amiodarone, amprenavir, atazanavir, cimetidine, indinavir, itraconazole, nelfinavir, ranitidine, ritonavir, saquinavir

Reactions

Skin
 Clammy skin (<1%)
 Diaphoresis (>10%) [3]
 Edema [1]
 Erythema (at application site) (<1%) [2]
 Exanthems
 Exfoliative dermatitis
 Fixed eruption [1]
 Papulo-nodular lesions (>1%)
 Pruritus (3–44%) [21]
 Purpura [1]
 Pustules (<1%)
 Rash (sic) (>1%) [2]
 Urticaria (<1%)

Cardiovascular
 Bradycardia [1]
 Flushing (3–10%)
 Hypotension [1]

Other
 Anaphylactoid reactions [4]
 Cough [2]
 Death [3]
 Dizziness [1]
 Dysesthesia (<1%)
 Dysgeusia (<1%)
 Headache
 Paresthesias (<1%)
 Xerostomia (>10%) [2]

FEVERFEW

Scientific names: *Chrysanthemum parthenium; Pyrethrum parthenium; Tanacetum parthenium*
Family: Asteraceae; Compositae
Trade and other common names: Atamisa; Featerfoiul; Featherfew; Featherfoil; MIG-99; Santa Maria
Category: Stimulant and tonic
Purported indications and other uses: Fever, headache, migraine, menstrual irregularities, arthritis, psoriasis, allergy, asthma, tinnitus, vertigo, nausea, cold, earache, orthopedic disorders, swollen feet, diarrhea, dyspepsia
Half-life: N/A
Clinically important, potentially hazardous interactions with: anticoagulants, NSAIDs, warfarin

Reactions

Skin
  Adverse effects (sic) (mild) [1]
  Allergic reactions (sic) [1]
  Angioedema (lips) [2]
  Dermatitis [2]
  Prurigo nodularis [1]

Other
  Ageusia [2]
  Bleeding [1]
  Oral ulceration [2]

FLUOXETINE

Trade names: Prozac (Lilly); Sarafem (Warner Chilcott)
Other common trade names: *Adofen; Apo-Fluoxetine; Dom-Fluoxetine; Fluctin; Fluctine; Fludac; Fluoxac; Fluoxeren; Fluxil; Fontex*
Indications: Depression, obsessive-compulsive disorder
Category: Antidepressant; Selective serotonin reuptake inhibitor (SSRI)
Half-life: 2–3 days
Clinically important, potentially hazardous interactions with: alprazolam, amphetamines, clarithromycin, clozapine, desipramine, dextroamphetamine, diethylpropion, duloxetine, erythromycin, haloperidol, imipramine, isocarboxazid, linezolid, lithium, MAO inhibitors, mazindol, meperidine, methamphetamine, midazolam, moclobemide, nortriptyline, phendimetrazine, phenelzine, phentermine, phenylpropanolamine, phenytoin, pimozide, pseudoephedrine, selegiline, serotonin agonists, sibutramine, **St John's wort**, sumatriptan, sympathomimetics, tramadol, tranylcypromine, trazodone, tricyclic antidepressants, troleandomycin, **tryptophan**

Reactions

Skin
  Acne (<1%)
  Allergic reactions (sic) [1]

  Angioedema [1]
  Bruising [1]
  Bullous eruption (<1%)

Candidiasis
Cellulitis
Dermatitis (<1%)
Diaphoresis (8.4%) [1]
Eczema (<1%)
Erythema multiforme [1]
Erythema nodosum (<1%)
Exanthems (4%) [7]
Exfoliative dermatitis
Facial edema (<1%)
Furunculosis (<1%)
Herpes simplex (reactivation) [1]
Herpes zoster
Lichenoid eruption
Lupus erythematosus (discoid)
Mycosis fungoides (exacerbation) [1]
Neuroleptic malignant syndrome [1]
Nodular eruption
Peripheral edema (<1%)
Petechiae (<1%)
Photosensitivity [1]
Phototoxicity (<1%) [2]
Pigmentation (<1%)
Pruritus (2.4%) [3]
Pseudo-mycosis fungoides [1]
Psoriasis (<1%) [1]
Purpura (<1%)
Pustules (<1%)
Rash (sic) (6%) [3]
Raynaud's phenomenon [1]
Seborrhea (<1%)
Stevens–Johnson syndrome [2]
Toxic epidermal necrolysis [2]
Ulcerations (<1%)
Urticaria (4%) [5]
Vasculitis [2]
Xerosis

Hair

Hair – alopecia (<1%) [10]
Hair – hirsutism (<1%)

Cardiovascular

Atrial fibrillation [1]
Bradycardia [1]
Flushing (<2%)
Hot flashes
QT prolongation [1]

Other

Ageusia (<1%)
Anaphylactoid reactions (<1%)
Aphthous stomatitis (<1%)
Black tongue [1]
Depression [1]
Dysgeusia (1.8%) [1]
Galactorrhea [1]
Gingivitis (<1%)
Glossitis (<1%)
Glossodynia [1]
Gynecomastia (<1%) [1]
Headache (<27%) [2]
Hyperesthesia (<1%)
Hypersensitivity [1]
Mastodynia (<1%)
Myalgia (<1%)
Oral ulceration (<1%) [1]
Paresthesias [2]
Parosmia (<1%)
Priapism (<1%)
Pseudolymphoma [3]
Rhabdomyolysis [1]
Serotonin syndrome [4]
Serum sickness [2]
Sialorrhea (<1%)
Stomatitis (<1%)
Thrombophlebitis (<1%)
Tinnitus
Tongue edema (<1%)
Tremor (2–10%)
Vaginal anesthesia [1]
Xerostomia (12%) [5]

FLUPHENAZINE

Trade name: Prolixin
Other common trade names: *Anatensol; Apo-Fluphenazine; Dapatum D25; Dapotum D; Fludecate; Modecate; Moditen*
Indications: Psychoses
Category: Phenothiazine antipsychotic
Half-life: 84–96 hours
Clinically important, potentially hazardous interactions with: antihistamines, arsenic, chlorpheniramine, dofetilide, **evening primrose**, quinolones, sparfloxacin

Reactions

Skin
Angioedema (<1%)
Dermatitis
Diaphoresis
Eczema
Edema
Erythema
Exanthems
Exfoliative dermatitis
Hypohidrosis (>10%)
Lupus erythematosus [1]
Peripheral edema
Photosensitivity
Pigmentation (<1%) (blue-gray) [1]
Pruritus (<1%)
Purpura
Rash (sic) (1–10%)
Seborrhea
Toxic epidermal necrolysis [1]
Urticaria
Vitiligo [2]
Xerosis

Other
Anaphylactoid reactions
Galactorrhea (1–10%)
Gynecomastia (1–10%)
Headache
Injection-site reactions
Mastodynia (1–10%)
Parkinsonism
Priapism (<1%) [2]
Rhabdomyolysis [1]
Sialorrhea [1]
Trembling (fingers)
Xerostomia (<1%)

FLURAZEPAM

Trade names: Dalmane (Valeant); Flurazepam (Watson)
Other common trade names: *Apo-Flurazepam; Benozil; Dalmadorm; Flunox; Nergart; Novoflupam; Som Pam; Somnol; Valdorm*
Indications: Insomnia
Category: Benzodiazepine sedative-hypnotic
Half-life: 40–114 hours
Clinically important, potentially hazardous interactions with: amprenavir, chlorpheniramine, clarithromycin, efavirenz, esomeprazole, imatinib, indinavir, nelfinavir, ritonavir

Reactions

Skin
Dermatitis (1–10%)
Diaphoresis (>10%)
Exanthems [1]
Pruritus
Purpura
Rash (sic) (>10%)
Urticaria

Cardiovascular
Flushing

Other
Acute intermittent porphyria
Dysgeusia (3.4%) (metallic taste) [1]
Headache
Oral lesions [1]
Paresthesias
Sialopenia (>10%)
Sialorrhea (1–10%)
Xerostomia (>10%)

FLUVOXAMINE

Trade name: Luvox (Solvay)
Other common trade names: *Apo-Fluvoxamine; Dumirox; Dumyrox; Faverin; Favoxil; Fevarin; Maveral*
Indications: Obsessive-compulsive disorder, depression
Category: Antidepressant; Selective serotonin reuptake inhibitor (SSRI)
Half-life: 15 hours
Clinically important, potentially hazardous interactions with: alprazolam, amphetamines, dextroamphetamine, diethylpropion, duloxetine, isocarboxazid, linezolid, MAO inhibitors, mazindol, methadone, methamphetamine, phendimetrazine, phenelzine, phentermine, phenylpropanolamine, pseudoephedrine, ropivacaine, selegiline, sibutramine, **St John's wort**, sumatriptan, sympathomimetics, tacrine, theophyllines, tramadol, tranylcypromine, trazodone, troleandomycin, **tryptophan**

Reactions

Skin
Acne (<1%)
Allergic reactions (sic) (<1%) [1]
Angioedema [1]
Bullous eruption
Dermatitis (<1%)
Diaphoresis (<7%) [1]
Edema (<1%)
Exanthems
Exfoliative dermatitis (<1%)
Furunculosis (<1%)
Neuroleptic malignant syndrome [1]
Photosensitivity (<1%) [2]
Pigmentation (<1%)
Pruritus
Purpura (<1%)
Rash (sic)
Seborrhea (<1%)
Stevens–Johnson syndrome
Toxic epidermal necrolysis (<1%) [1]
Urticaria (<1%)
Xerosis (<1%)

Hair
Hair – alopecia (<1%)
Hair – alopecia areata [1]

Hematopoietic
Ecchymoses (<1%)

Other

Ageusia (<1%)
Anaphylactoid reactions
Dysgeusia (3%)
Fatigue [1]
Gingivitis (<1%)
Glossitis (<1%)
Headache
Hyperactivity [1]
Mastodynia (<1%)

Myalgia (<1%)
Oral lesions (10%) [1]
Paresthesias
Parosmia (<1%)
Priapism
Serotonin syndrome [3]
Sialorrhea
Stomatitis (<1%)
Vaginitis (<1%) [1]
Xerostomia (<14%) [1]

FOSPHENYTOIN

Trade name: Cerebyx (Eisai)
Indications: Seizure prophylaxis, status epilepticus
Category: Anticonvulsant
Half-life: 15 minutes
Clinically important, potentially hazardous interactions with: chloramphenicol, cyclosporine, disulfiram, dopamine, imatinib, itraconazole

Fosphenytoin is a prodrug of phenytoin

Reactions

Skin

Acne (<1%)
Bullous eruption [1]
Chills
Erythema multiforme (<1%) [1]
Exanthems
Exfoliative dermatitis (<1%) [1]
Facial edema
Lupus erythematosus [1]
Pruritus (48.9%) [4]
Rash (sic) (<1%)
Stevens–Johnson syndrome
Toxic epidermal necrolysis

Hematopoietic

Ecchymoses

Other

Application-site pain [1]
Dysgeusia (3.3%)
Gingival hypertrophy [1]
Headache
Hyperesthesia (2.2%)
Paresthesias (4.4%) [2]
Tongue disorder (sic)
Xerostomia (4.4%)

FROVATRIPTAN

Trade name: Frova (Vernalis)
Indications: Migraine headaches
Category: 5-HT1 (serotonin) receptor agonist; Antimigraine
Half-life: 26 hours

Reactions

Skin
  Bullous eruption (<1%)
  Cheilitis (<1%)
  Diaphoresis (1%)
  Pruritus (<1%)
  Purpura (<1%)
  Rash (sic)

Eyes
  Conjunctivitis (<1%)

Cardiovascular
  Flushing (4%)
  Hot flashes (<1%)

Other
  Arthralgia (<1%)
  Bone or joint pain (3%)

Depression (<1%)
Dysesthesia (1%)
Dysgeusia (<1%)
Headache
Hyperesthesia (<1%)
Myalgia (<1%)
Pain (1%)
Paresthesias (4%) [1]
Sialopenia (3%)
Sialorrhea (<1%)
Stomatitis (<1%)
Tinnitus (1%)
Toothache (1%)
Tremor (<1%)
Xerostomia

GABAPENTIN

Trade name: Neurontin (Pfizer)
Indications: Seizures
Category: Anticonvulsant
Half-life: 5–6 hours

Reactions

Skin
  Acne (>1%)
  Acute febrile neutrophilic dermatosis
    (Sweet's syndrome) [2]
  Anticonvulsant hypersensitivity syndrome
    [1]
  Bullous pemphigoid [1]
  Edema [3]
  Exanthems [2]
  Facial edema (<1%)

Peripheral edema (1.7%) [2]
Pruritus (1.3%)
Purpura (<1%) [1]
Rash (sic) (>1%)
Stevens–Johnson syndrome [1]
Urticaria
Vasculitis

Hair
  Hair – alopecia [1]

Other
Ataxia [1]
Dizziness [3]
Foetor ex ore (halitosis) [1]
Gingivitis (<1%)
Glossitis
Gynecomastia [1]
Myalgia (2%)
Myoclonus [1]
Paresthesias (<1%)
Priapism [1]
Sialorrhea
Stomatitis
Tinnitus
Tooth pigmentation
Tremor (1–10%) [1]
Xerostomia (1.7%)

GALANTAMINE

Trade name: Reminyl (Janssen)
Indications: Alzheimer's disease
Category: Acetylcholinesterase inhibitor
Half-life: 6–8 hours
Clinically important, potentially hazardous interactions with: bethanechol, cimetidine, donepezil, edrophonium, physostigmine, pilocarpine, rivastigmine, succinylcholine, tacrine

Note: Derived from snowdrop (*Galanthus* sp) bulbs

Reactions

Skin
Acute generalized exanthematous
    pustulosis (AGEP) [1]
Edema
Peripheral edema (>2%)
Purpura (>2%)
Upper respiratory infection (>2%)

Cardiovascular
QT prolongation [1]

Other
Depression (5%) [1]
Headache [1]
Paresthesias [1]
Sialorrhea
Tremor (1–10%)
Xerostomia

GINKGO BILOBA

Scientific name: *Ginkgo biloba (Mericon)*
Family: Ginkgoaceae
Trade and other common names: Fossil Tree; Japanese Silver Apricot; Maidenhair Tree; Salisburia; Tanakan; Tebonin
Category: Antidementia; Improved cognition
Purported indications and other uses: Dementia, memory loss, headache, tinnitus, dizziness, mood disturbances, hearing disorders, intermittent claudication, attention deficit hyperactivity disorder, premenstrual syndrome, heart disease
Half-life: N/A
Clinically important, potentially hazardous interactions with: anticoagulants, aspirin, diuretics, NSAIDs, phenytoin, platelet inhibitors, SSRIs, **St John's wort**, thiazide diuretics, trazodone, warfarin

Reactions

Skin
Adverse effects (sic) [3]
Allergic reactions (sic)
Dermatitis [2]
Erythema
Exanthems [1]
Pruritus
Rash (sic)
Vasculitis
Vesiculation

Eyes
Hyphema [1]

Other
Phlebitis
Rectal burning
Seizures [4]
Spontaneous bleeding [12]
Stomatitis

Note: *Ginkgo biloba* is the oldest living tree species in the world. Ginkgo is the most frequently prescribed herbal medicine in Germany

GINSENG

Scientific name: *Panax ginseng*
Family: Araliaceae
Trade and other common names: Asian Ginseng; Asiatic Ginseng; Chinese Ginseng; Japanese Ginseng; Jintsam; Korean Ginseng; Korean Red; Ninjin; Red Ginseng; Ren She; Sang; Seng
Category: Immune stimulant
Purported indications and other uses: General tonic, improving stamina, cognitive function, concentration, diuretic, antidepressant, gastritis, neurasthenia, impotence, fever, hangover, cancer, cardiovascular diseases
Half-life: N/A
Clinically important, potentially hazardous interactions with: alcohol, aspirin, **caffeine**, digoxin, olmesartan, phenelzine, tamoxifen, ticlopidine, warfarin

Reactions

Skin
  Adverse effects (sic) [3]
  Allergic reactions (sic)
  Burning (sensation) [1]
  Edema
  Pruritus
  Stevens–Johnson syndrome [2]

Other
  Bleeding [4]
  Gynecomastia [1]
  Mastodynia [3]
  Penile pain
  Side effects (sic) [1]

Note: Ginseng has been used for medicinal purposes for more than 2000 years. Approximately 6,000,000 Americans use it regularly

GREEN TEA

Scientific names: *Camellia sinensis; Camellia thea; Camellia theifera; Thea bohea; Thea sinensis; Thea viridis*
Family: Theaceae
Trade and other common names: Chinese tea
Category: Astringent; Improved cognition
Purported indications and other uses: Improving cognitive performance, stomach disorders, nausea, vomiting, diarrhea, anticancer, headaches, Crohn's disease. **Topical**: soothe sunburn, bleeding gums, reduce sweating
Half-life: N/A
Clinically important, potentially hazardous interactions with: warfarin

Note: Tea is consumed as a beverage

Reactions

None

HALOPERIDOL

Trade name: Haldol (Ortho-McNeil)
Other common trade names: *Dozic; Duraperidol; Haloper; Peridol; Seranace; Serenace*
Indications: Psychoses, Tourette's disorder
Category: Phenothiazine antipsychotic; Sedative
Half-life: 20 hours
Clinically important, potentially hazardous interactions with: eucalyptus, fluoxetine, lithium, methotrexate, propranolol

Reactions

Skin

Acne
Cellulitis [1]
Dermatitis (<1%)
Diaphoresis [1]
Exanthems
Exfoliative dermatitis
Neuroleptic malignant syndrome [6]
Pemphigus foliaceus [1]
Photo-recall [1]
Photosensitivity (<1%) [3]
Pigmentation (<1%)
Pruritus (<1%)
Purpura
Rash (sic) (<1%)
Seborrheic dermatitis [2]
Urticaria

Hair

Hair – alopecia (<1%) [1]
Hair – alopecia areata [2]
Hair – depigmentation [1]

Cardiovascular

Flushing [1]
QT prolongation [1]
Torsades de pointes [2]
Torsades de pointes [1]

Other

Akathisia [2]
Death [4]
Galactorrhea (<1%)
Gynecomastia (<1%)
Headache
Injection-site hypersensitivity [1]
Injection-site pain [1]
Injection-site reactions (sic) [3]
Mastodynia
Parkinsonism (pseudo) [1]
Priapism (<1%)
Rhabdomyolysis [2]
Sialorrhea [1]
Tardive dyskinesia (<37%) [1]
Tremor [1]
Xerostomia (<1%) [2]

HEROIN

Trade name: Heroin
Indications: Recreational drug
Category: Diacetylmorphine; Semisynthetic narcotic; Substance abuse drug
Half-life: N/A

Reactions

Skin
Abscess [7]
Acanthosis nigricans [2]
Acne [1]
Angioedema [1]
Bullous impetigo [1]
Burning (24%) [1]
Candidiasis [3]
Cellulitis [3]
Dermatitis [1]
Ecthyma [1]
Ecthyma gangrenosum [1]
Edema [4]
Exanthems [2]
Excoriations [1]
Fixed eruption [2]
Folliculitis (candidal) [4]
Glucagonoma syndrome (necrolytic migratory erythema) [1]
Infections (13%) [1]
Kaposi's sarcoma [1]
Necrosis [3]
Necrotizing fasciitis [1]
Pemphigus [1]
Pemphigus erythematodes [1]
Pemphigus vegetans [1]
Perforating collagenosis [1]
Photosensitivity [2]

Pigmentation [4]
Pruritus [6]
Purpura [1]
Pustules [5]
Side effects (sic) (85%)
Toxic epidermal necrolysis [2]
Ulcerations [4]
Urticaria [3]
Vasculitis [2]
Vesiculation (arms) [1]

Eyes
Eyelid edema [2]

Other
Death [4]
Hypersensitivity [1]
Injection-site scarring [1]
Injection-site ulceration [3]
Myalgia [1]
Necrotizing vasculitis (tongue) [1]
Oral ulceration (tongue) [1]
Polyarteritis nodosa [1]
Rhabdomyolysis [9]
Seizures (2%) [1]
Serum sickness [1]
Sweat gland necrosis [1]
Tongue pigmentation (fixed eruption) [1]
Tooth decay [1]

HYDROXYZINE

Trade names: Atarax (Pfizer); Marax; Vistaril (Pfizer)
Other common trade names: *AH3 N; Anaxanil; Bobsule; Iremofar; Masmoran; Multipax; Otarex; Paxistil; Quiess; Rezine; Vamate*
Indications: Anxiety and tension, pruritus
Category: Antihistamine; Anxiolytic
Half-life: 3–7 hours
Clinically important, potentially hazardous interactions with: alcohol, barbiturates, CNS depressants, narcotics, non-narcotic analgesics

Reactions

Skin
  Angioedema (<1%) [3]
  Dermatitis [1]
  Diaphoresis
  Edema (<1%)
  Erythema multiforme (<1%) [1]
  Exanthems [3]
  Fixed eruption [3]
  Photosensitivity (<1%)
  Purpura
  Rash (sic) (<1%)

Urticaria [2]

Cardiovascular
  Flushing [1]

Other
  Hypersensitivity [1]
  Injection-site necrosis [1]
  Myalgia (<1%)
  Priapism [1]
  Xerostomia (12%) [2]

HYOSCYAMINE

Synonyms: Hyoscyamine sulfate; hyoscyamine sulfate
Trade names: Anaspaz; Cytospaz; Donnamar; ED-SPAZ; Gastrosed; Hyco; Hycosol SI; Hyospaz; IB-Stat (InKline); Levbid (Schwarz); Levsin (Schwarz); Levsin/SL (Schwarz); Levsinex (Schwarz); Medispaz; Nulev (Schwarz); Pasmex; Setamine; Urised
Other common trade names: *Duboisine; Egacene Durettes; Egazil; Peptard*
Indications: Treatment of gastrointestinal tract disorders caused by spasm, Adjunctive therapy for peptic ulcers, cystitis, parkinsonism, biliary & renal colic
Category: Anticholinergic
Duration of action: 13–38 min
Clinically important, potentially hazardous interactions with: anticholinergics, arbutamine

Reactions

Skin
  Allergic reactions (sic)
  Hypohidrosis (>10%)
  Photosensitivity (1–10%)
  Rash (sic) (<1%)

Urticaria
Xerosis (>10%)

Cardiovascular
  Flushing

Other
 Ageusia
 Anaphylactoid reactions
 Dysgeusia

Headache
Injection-site inflammation (>10%)
Xerostomia (>10%)

IMIPRAMINE

Trade name: Tofranil (Mallinckrodt) (Novartis)
Other common trade names: Apo-Imipramine; Imidol; Imipramin; Impril; Novo-Pramine; Primonil; Pryleugan
Indications: Depression
Category: Tricyclic antidepressant
Half-life: 6–18 hours
Clinically important, potentially hazardous interactions with: amprenavir, arbutamine, clonidine, epinephrine, fluoxetine, formoterol, guanethidine, isocarboxazid, linezolid, MAO inhibitors, phenelzine, quinolones, sparfloxacin, tranylcypromine

Reactions

Skin
 Acne
 Allergic reactions (sic)
 Angioedema (<1%) [1]
 Bullous eruption [1]
 Diaphoresis (1–25%) [7]
 Edema [1]
 Erythema
 Exanthems (1–6%) [6]
 Exfoliative dermatitis [4]
 Fixed eruption (<1%) [1]
 Lichen planus [1]
 Lupus erythematosus [1]
 Peripheral edema
 Petechiae
 Photosensitivity (<1%) [3]
 Pigmentation [9]
 Pruritus (3%) [6]
 Purpura [3]
 Rash (sic)
 Urticaria [6]
 Vasculitis [1]
 Xerosis

Hair
 Hair – alopecia (<1%) [2]
 Hair – alopecia areata [1]

Nails
 Nails – parrot-beak [1]

Cardiovascular
 Bradycardia [1]
 Flushing [1]
 QT prolongation [1]
 Tachycardia [1]

Other
 Black tongue
 Dysgeusia (>10%) (metallic taste) [1]
 Galactorrhea (<1%) [1]
 Glossitis [2]
 Glossodynia
 Gynecomastia (<1%) [1]
 Hypogeusia
 Mucous membrane desquamation [1]
 Oral lesions [3]
 Oral ulceration
 Paresthesias
 Parkinsonism (1–10%)
 Stomatitis [2]
 Tremor
 Vaginitis
 Xerostomia (>10%) [5]

ISOCARBOXAZID

Trade name: Marplan (Oxford)
Other common trade name: *Enerzer*
Indications: Depression
Category: Antidepressant; Monoamine oxidase (MAO) inhibitor
Half-life: N/A
Clinically important, potentially hazardous interactions with: amitriptyline, amoxapine, bupropion, citalopram, clomipramine, desipramine, doxepin, fluoxetine, fluvoxamine, imipramine, meperidine, nefazodone, nortriptyline, paroxetine, protriptyline, rizatriptan, sertraline, sibutramine, sumatriptan, trimipramine, **tryptophan**, venlafaxine, zolmitriptan

Reactions

Skin
Diaphoresis [1]
Exanthems (7%) [1]
Peripheral edema (1–10%)
Photosensitivity (4%) [1]
Pruritus (4%) [1]

Rash (sic)
Telangiectasia

Other
Black tongue
Xerostomia (1–10%) [1]

KAVA

Scientific name: *Piper methysticum*
Family: Piperaceae
Trade and other common names: Ava; Awa; Intoxicating Pepper; Kavosporal; Kew; Sakau; Tonga
Category: Anxiolytic; Sedative
Purported indications and other uses: Psychosis, depression, headache, migraines, colds, rheumatism, cystitis, vaginal prolapse, otitis, abscesses, antistress, analgesic, local anesthetic, anticonvulsant
Half-life: N/A
Clinically important, potentially hazardous interactions with: alcohol, alprazolam, benzodiazepines, escitalopram, levodopa

Note: Products containing kava have been implicated in cases of severe liver toxicity. Serious adverse effects include hepatitis, cirrhosis and liver failure. At least one patient required a liver transplant. Kava has now been banned in many countries

Reactions

Skin
Adverse effects (sic) [6]
Dermopathy (pellagra-like syndrome) [3]
Lymphocytic inflammation of the dermis
Photosensitivity

Pigmentation (yellow)
Pruritus
Rash (sic)
Scaly dermatitis
Seborrheic dermatitis [1]

Xerosis
Hair
  Hair – pigmentation

Nails
  Nails – pigmentation

Other
  Death [1]

Dizziness [1]
Hypersensitivity [1]
Mouth numbness
Parkinsonism [1]
Seizures [1]
Side effects (sic) [3]

Note: Kava was discovered by Captain Cook, who named the plant 'intoxicating pepper.' In the South Pacific, kava is a popular social drink, similar to alcohol in Western societies

KETAMINE

Trade name: Ketalar (Monarch)
Other common trade names: *Calypsol; Ketalin; Ketanest; Ketolar; Petar*
Indications: Induction of anesthesia
Category: Anesthetic; Sedative-hypnotic
Half-life: 2–3 hours
Clinically important, potentially hazardous interactions with: memantine

Reactions

Skin
  Erythema
  Exanthems
  Pruritus [2]
  Rash (sic) (1–10%)

Cardiovascular
  Bradycardia [1]

Other
  Injection-site erythema
  Injection-site pain (1–10%)
  Sialorrhea (<1%) [1]
  Tremor (>10%)

L-CARNITINE

Trade names: Aplegin; L-Carnipure
Other common trade names: *Acetyl-L-carnitine; B(t)Factor; Carnitine; Carnitor; Levocarnitine; Propionyl-L-carnitine; Vitacarn; Vitamin B(t)*
Indications: Improves lipid metabolism, red blood cell count, and antioxidant status, chronic fatigue syndrome, dementia, angina, post-MI cardioprotection, congestive heart failure, valproate toxicity, anorexia
Category: Dietary supplement

Note: Mixed D, L-carnitine has been associated with myasthenic syndrome.

Reactions

None

LAMOTRIGINE

Synonyms: BW-430C; LTG
Trade name: Lamictal (GSK)
Indications: Epilepsy
Category: Anticonvulsant
Half-life: 24 hours
Clinically important, potentially hazardous interactions with: oral contraceptives

Reactions

Skin

Acne (1.3%)
Acute generalized exanthematous
 pustulosis (AGEP) [1]
Adverse effects (sic) [1]
Angioedema (1–10%) [1]
Anticonvulsant hypersensitivity syndrome
 [5]
Bullous eruption [1]
Diaphoresis (<1%)
Eczema (<1%)
Erythema (1–10%) [1]
Erythema multiforme [3]
Exanthems (1–10%) [12]
Facial edema (<1%)
Fixed eruption [1]
Flu-like syndrome (7%)
Hyperhidrosis [1]
Lupus erythematosus [1]
Petechiae (<1%)
Photosensitivity [2]
Pruritus (3.1%) [1]
Rash (sic) (10–20%) [24]
Stevens–Johnson syndrome (1–10%) [20]
Toxic epidermal necrolysis [26]
Urticaria (<1%)
Xerosis (<1%)

Hair

Hair – alopecia (1.3%)
Hair – hirsutism (<1%)

Hematopoietic

Ecchymoses (<1%)

Cardiovascular

Flushing (<1%)
Hot flashes (1–10%)

Other

Anaphylactoid reactions [1]
Death
Dizziness [1]
Dysgeusia (<1%) [1]
Foetor ex ore (halitosis) (<1%)
Gingival hypertrophy (<1%)
Gingivitis (<1%)
Headache [1]
Hyperesthesia (<1%)
Hypersensitivity (1–10%) [17]
Lymphadenopathy [1]
Myalgia (>1%)
Oral ulceration (<1%)
Paresthesias (>1%)
Porphyria [1]
Pseudolymphoma [1]
Sialorrhea (<1%)
Stomatitis (<1%)
Tic disorder [1]
Tremor [4]
Vaginitis (4.1%)
Vulvovaginal candidiasis (<1%)
Xerostomia (1%)

LAVENDER

Scientific names: *Lavandula angustifolia; Lavandula dentata; Lavandula spica; Lavandula vera*
Family: Lamiaceae
Trade and other common names: Alhucema; English Lavender; French Lavender; Spanish Lavender; Spike Lavender
Category: Sedative
Purported indications and other uses: Restlessness, insomnia, loss of appetite, flatulence, colic, giddiness, nervous headache, migraine, toothache, sprains, neuralgia, rheumatism, acne, pimples, nausea, vomiting. Flavoring, fragrance, insect repellent
Half-life: N/A

Reactions

Skin
  Dermatitis [2]

LEMON BALM

Scientific name: *Melissa officinalis*
Family: Labiatae
Trade and other common names: Balm mint; Blue balm; Dropsy plant; Garden balm; Melissa; Pharmaton; Sweet balm
Category: Antibacterial; Antispasmodic; Antiviral; Carminative; Mild sedative
Purported indications and other uses: Oral: Alzheimer's disease, anxiety, attention deficit disorder, colic, dementia, depression, hyperactivity, hyperthyroidism, insomnia, menstrual cramps, fevers, headache. **Topical:** genital herpes, herpes simplex, insect bites, insect repellent, muscle tension, skin irritation
Half-life: N/A

Reactions

None

LEVETIRACETAM

Trade name: Keppra (UCB Pharma)
Indications: Partial onset seizures
Category: Anticonvulsant
Half-life: 7 hours

Reactions

Skin   Flu-like syndrome [1]
  Edema [1]   Fungal dermatitis (>1%)

Infections (sic) (13–26%) [5]
Rash (sic) (>1%)

Hematopoietic
Ecchymoses (<1%)

Other
Asthenia (<22%) [3]

Dizziness (9–18%) [4]
Gingivitis (>1%)
Headache (25%) [1]
Pain [1]
Paresthesias (2%)

LITHIUM

Trade names: Eskalith (GSK); Lithobid (Solvay); Lithonate; Lithotabs
Other common trade names: Carbolith; Duralith; Hynorex Retard; Lithicarb; Lithizine; Priadel; Teralithe
Indications: Manic-depressive states
Category: Antidepressant; Antipsychotic
Half-life: 18–24 hours
Clinically important, potentially hazardous interactions with: acetazolamide, acitretin, bendroflumethiazide, benzthiazide, chlorothiazide, chlorthalidone, fluoxetine, **guarana**, haloperidol, hydrochlorothiazide, hydroflumethiazide, indapamide, meperidine, methotrexate, methyclothiazide, metolazone, olmesartan, pegfilgrastim, polythiazide, quinethazone, rofecoxib, sibutramine, thiazides*, trichlormethiazide, valdecoxib

Note: An excellent review of the cutaneous conditions associated with lithium can be found in (1983): Sarantidis D+, Br J Psychiatry 143, 42

Reactions

Skin
Acanthosis nigricans [1]
Acne [16]
Angioedema [2]
Angular cheilitis (1%) [1]
Atopic dermatitis (3%) [1]
Bullous eruption [1]
Darier's disease [3]
Dermatitis [4]
Dermatitis herpetiformis [3]
Discoloration of fingers and toes (<1%)
Eczema [1]
Edema [3]
Erythema [1]
Erythema multiforme [1]
Exanthems [9]
Exfoliative dermatitis (1%) [3]
Follicular keratosis [3]
Folliculitis [4]

Hidradenitis [4]
Hyperplasia (verrucous) [1]
Ichthyosis (1%) [2]
Keratoderma [1]
Keratosis pilaris [2]
Lichen planus [1]
Lichen simplex chronicus [1]
Linear IgA dermatosis [4]
Lupus erythematosus [4]
Morphea [1]
Mycosis fungoides [1]
Myxedema [10]
Neuroleptic malignant syndrome [2]
Papulo-nodular lesions (elbows) [2]
Port-wine stain [1]
Prurigo nodularis (1%) [1]
Pruritus (<1%) [8]
Psoriasis (2%) [45]
Purpura [2]

Pustular psoriasis [3]
Pustules [2]
Rash (sic) (1–10%) [1]
Seborrheic dermatitis [3]
Side effects (sic) (23–33%) [3]
Subcorneal pustular dermatosis (Sneddon–Wilkinson) [1]
Telangiectasia [1]
Tinea [1]
Toxicoderma [1]
Ulcerations (lower extremities) [5]
Urticaria [3]
Vasculitis [4]
Verrucous lesions [1]
Warts [1]
Xerosis [1]

Hair
Hair – alopecia (10–19%) [17]
Hair – alopecia areata (2%) [3]
Hair – brittle [1]
Hair – changes in texture [1]

Nails
Nails – Beau's lines (transverse nail bands) [1]
Nails – dystrophy [2]
Nails – onychomadesis [1]
Nails – psoriasis [1]

Cardiovascular
Bradycardia [1]
Cardiomegaly [1]
ECG changes (abnormalities) [1]
QT prolongation [1]

Other
Dysgeusia (>10%)
Fever [1]
Geographic tongue [1]
Gingival hypertrophy [1]
Glossodynia
Headache
Lichenoid stomatitis [3]
Oral ulceration [3]
Parkinsonism [1]
Pseudolymphoma [1]
Pseudotumor cerebri (<1%)
Rhabdomyolysis [2]
Sialorrhea
Stomatitis [2]
Stomatodynia [1]
Stutter [1]
Tinnitus
Tremor
Vaginal ulceration [1]
Xerostomia (<1%) [1]

LORAZEPAM

Trade name: Ativan (Wyeth) (Baxter)
Other common trade names: *Apo-Lorazepam; Durazolam; Laubeel; Merlit; Nu-Loraz; Punktyl; Tavor; Temesta; Titus*
Indications: Anxiety, depression
Category: Anticonvulsant; Antiemetic; Benzodiazepine anxiolytic
Half-life: 10–20 hours
Clinically important, potentially hazardous interactions with: alcohol, amprenavir, barbiturates, chlorpheniramine, clarithromycin, CNS depressants, efavirenz, erythromycin, esomeprazole, imatinib, MAO inhibitors, narcotics, nelfinavir, phenothiazines, valproate

Reactions

Skin
Dermatitis (1–10%)
Diaphoresis (>10%)
Erythema multiforme [1]
Exanthems
Fixed eruption [1]
Pruritus
Purpura
Rash (sic) (>10%)
Stevens–Johnson syndrome [1]
Urticaria

Hair
Hair – alopecia
Hair – hirsutism

Cardiovascular
Bradycardia [1]
Hypotension [1]

Other
Gingival lichenoid reaction [1]
Headache
Injection-site pain (>10%) [1]
Injection-site phlebitis (>10%) [1]
Paresthesias
Pseudolymphoma [2]
Rhabdomyolysis [1]
Sialopenia (>10%)
Sialorrhea (<1%) [1]
Tremor (1–10%)
Xerostomia (>10%)

LOXAPINE

Trade name: Loxitane (Watson)
Other common trade names: *Desconex; Loxapac*
Indications: Psychoses
Category: Anxiolytic; Tricyclic antipsychotic
Half-life: 12–19 hours (terminal)

Reactions

Skin
Dermatitis [1]
Diaphoresis
Exanthems
Facial edema
Neuroleptic malignant syndrome [1]
Photosensitivity (<1%) [1]
Pigmentation (<1%)
Pruritus (<1%) [1]
Purpura
Rash (sic) (1–10%)
Seborrhea [1]
Side effects (sic)
Urticaria

Hair
Hair – alopecia

Other
Galactorrhea (<1%)
Gynecomastia (1–10%)
Headache
Myalgia [1]
Paresthesias
Parkinsonism
Priapism (<1%)
Rhabdomyolysis [1]
Xerostomia (>10%)

MAPROTILINE

Trade name: Ludiomil (Novartis)
Other common trade names: *Delgian; Maprostad; Melodil; Mirpan; Nono-Maprotiline; Psymion; Retinyl*
Indications: Depression, anxiety
Category: Tetracyclic antidepressant
Half-life: 27–58 hours

Reactions

Skin
  Acne [3]
  Diaphoresis (3–8%) [1]
  Edema
  Erythema
  Erythema multiforme [1]
  Exanthems (1–9%) [3]
  Ichthyosis [1]
  Petechiae
  Photosensitivity [2]
  Pruritus
  Purpura [1]
  Rash (sic) (>10%)
  Stevens–Johnson syndrome [1]
  Urticaria (4%) [2]
  Vasculitis [1]

Hair
  Hair – alopecia [2]

Cardiovascular
  Flushing
  Torsades de pointes [1]

Other
  Black tongue
  Dysgeusia
  Galactorrhea
  Gynecomastia (<1%)
  Headache
  Parkinsonism
  Sialorrhea
  Stomatitis
  Tinnitus
  Tremor
  Xerostomia (20–40%) [1]

MARIHUANA

Trade name: Marihuana
Indications: Nausea and vomiting, substance abuse drug
Category: Hallucinogen
Half-life: N/A
Clinically important, potentially hazardous interactions with: atazanavir

Note: Marihuana is the popular name for the dried flowering leaves of the hemp plant, *Cannabis sativa*. It contains tetrahydrocannabinols. It is also known as 'pot,' 'grass,' 'hashish,' etc

Reactions

Skin
  Allergic reactions (sic) [1]
  Exanthems
  Pruritus

Squamous metaplasia [1]
Urticaria

Cardiovascular
  Angina [1]
  Bradycardia [1]
  Chest pain [1]
  Hypotension [1]

Other
  Anaphylactoid reactions [1]
  Death [1]

MDMA*

Trade name: Ecstacy
Indications: N/A
Category: Hallucinogenic 'designer drug'; Psychotherapeutic; Recreational drug
Half-life: N/A

Reactions

Skin
  Acne [1]
  Chills
  Diaphoresis [3]
  Neuroleptic malignant syndrome [1]
  Rash (sic)

Cardiovascular
  Congestive heart failure [1]
  Flushing [1]

Other
  Bruxism [2]

Death [38]
Depression (37%) [8]
Jaw clenching [2]
Myalgia
Oral ulceration [1]
Paresthesias [1]
Parkinsonism [4]
Priapism [1]
Rhabdomyolysis [24]
Serotonin syndrome [2]
Tremor
Xerostomia [1]

*Note: 3,4-Methylenedioxymethamphetamine

MECLIZINE

Trade name: Antivert (Pfizer)
Other common trade names: *Antrizine; Bonamine; Bonine; Dizmiss; Dramamine II; Dramine; Meni-D; Nico-Vert; Peremesin; Postadoxin; Postafen; Suprimal; Vergon*
Indications: Motion sickness
Category: Antiemetic; Antihistamine H_1-blocker
Half-life: 6 hours
Clinically important, potentially hazardous interactions with: alcohol, barbiturates, chloral hydrate, ethchlorvynol, paraldehyde, phenothiazines, zolpidem

Reactions

Skin
  Angioedema (<1%)

Exanthems [1]
Photosensitivity (<1%)

Rash (sic) (<1%)
Urticaria

Other
Myalgia (<1%)

Paresthesias (<1%)
Tremor
Xerostomia (1–10%)

MELATONIN

Scientific name: *N-acetyl-5-methoxytryptamine*
Family: None
Trade and other common names: MEL; MLT
Category: Chemoprotectant; Circadian rhythm regulator
Purported indications and other uses: Jet lag, sleep disorders, Alzheimer's disease, free radical scavenger, chemotherapy adjunct, tinnitus, depression, migraine, cluster headache, hypertension, hyperpigmentation, osteoporosis, antioxidant. Skin protectant against sunburn
Half-life: N/A
Clinically important, potentially hazardous interactions with: acetaminophen, NSAIDs, warfarin, zoloft

Reactions

Skin
Fixed eruption [2]
Photosensitivity [1]

Other
Crohn's disease [1]
Seizures [1]

MEMANTINE

Trade name: Namenda (Forest)
Indications: Alzheimer's disease, Vascular dementia
Category: NMDA receptor antagonist
Half-life: 60–80 hours
Clinically important, potentially hazardous interactions with: amantadine, dextromethorphan, ketamine

Reactions

Skin
Allergic reactions (sic) (<1%)
Cellulitis (<1%)
Dermatitis (<1%)
Eczema (<1%)
Exanthems (<1%)
Flu-like syndrome (>2%)
Peripheral edema (>2%)

Pruritus (<1%)
Rash (sic) (>1%)
Ulcerations (<1%)
Urticaria (<1%)

Hair
Hair – alopecia (<1%)

Eyes
  Blepharitis

Other
  Abdominal pain [1]
  Arthralgia (>2%)
  Back pain (3%)

Cough (4%)
Depression (>2%)
Dizziness (7%) [2]
Fatigue (2%)
Headache (6%)
Tinnitus

MEPHENYTOIN

Trade name: Mesantoin (Novartis)
Other common trade names: *Epilan-Gerot; Epilanex*
Indications: Partial seizures
Category: Hydantoin anticonvulsant
Half-life: 7 hours (for the active metabolite: 95–144 hours)
Clinically important, potentially hazardous interactions with: chloramphenicol, cyclosporine, disulfiram, dopamine, imatinib, itraconazole

Reactions

Skin
  Acne [1]
  Angioedema [1]
  Bullous eruption [1]
  Dermatomyositis [1]
  Edema
  Erythema multiforme [3]
  Exanthems (8–10%) [5]
  Exfoliative dermatitis [1]
  Lupus erythematosus [11]
  Pigmentation [4]
  Pruritus [1]
  Purpura [1]

Scleroderma [1]
Side effects (sic) [1]
Stevens–Johnson syndrome [1]
Toxic epidermal necrolysis [4]
Urticaria [3]

Hair
  Hair – alopecia

Other
  Gingival hypertrophy
  Oral mucosal eruption [1]
  Polyarteritis nodosa [1]
  Stomatitis [1]

MEPHOBARBITAL

Trade name: Mebaral
Other common trade name: *Prominal*
Indications: Epilepsy, anxiety
Category: Anticonvulsant; Barbiturate ; Sedative
Half-life: 34 hours
Clinically important, potentially hazardous interactions with: alcohol, anticoagulants, antihistamines, brompheniramine, buclizine, chlorpheniramine, dicumarol, ethanolamine, imatinib, warfarin

Reactions

Skin
  Angioedema (<1%)
  Exanthems
  Exfoliative dermatitis (<1%)
  Purpura
  Rash (sic) (<1%)
  Stevens–Johnson syndrome (<1%)

  Urticaria
Other
  Rhabdomyolysis [1]
  Serum sickness
  Thrombophlebitis (<1%)

MEPROBAMATE

Trade names: Equagesic (Women First); Miltown (MedPointe)
Other common trade names: *Harmonin; Meditran; Meditrara; Meprate; Meprospan; Miltaun; Neuramate; Praol; Probamyl; Urbilat; Visanon*
Indications: Anxiety, insomnia
Category: Anxiolytic
Half-life: 10 hours

Reactions

Skin
  Allergic reactions (sic) [1]
  Angioedema (<1%) [4]
  Bullous eruption (<1%) [2]
  Dermatitis (<1%)
  Eczema [1]
  Erythema multiforme (<1%) [2]
  Erythema nodosum (<1%)
  Exanthems (2%) [11]
  Exfoliative dermatitis
  Fixed eruption (<1%) [5]
  Lupus erythematosus [1]
  Pemphigus foliaceus [1]

  Peripheral edema (<1%)
  Petechiae [1]
  Photosensitivity [1]
  Pityriasis rosea [1]
  Pruritus (<1%) [6]
  Purpura (<1%) [13]
  Rash (sic) (1–10%)
  Side effects (sic) (2%) [2]
  Stevens–Johnson syndrome (<1%) [2]
  Toxic epidermal necrolysis (<1%) [1]
  Toxic erythema [1]
  Urticaria (2%) [10]
  Vasculitis [8]

Hematopoietic
Ecchymoses

Other
Acute intermittent porphyria [1]
Anaphylactoid reactions [1]
Gynecomastia
Headache
Hypersensitivity

Oral mucosal eruption [1]
Oral ulceration
Paresthesias
Polyarteritis nodosa [1]
Porphyria [1]
Rhabdomyolysis [1]
Stomatitis (<1%) [1]
Xerostomia

MESORIDAZINE

Trade name: Serentil (Boehringer Ingelheim)
Other common trade name: *Mesorin*
Indications: Schizophrenia
Category: Phenothiazine antipsychotic
Half-life: 24–48 hours
Clinically important, potentially hazardous interactions with: antihistamines, arsenic, chlorpheniramine, dofetilide, piperazine, quinolones, sparfloxacin, telithromycin

Reactions

Skin
Angioedema
Dermatitis
Eczema
Edema
Erythema
Exfoliative dermatitis
Hypohidrosis (>10%)
Lupus erythematosus
Peripheral edema
Photosensitivity (1–10%)
Pigmentation (blue-gray) (<1%)
Pruritus
Rash (sic) (1–10%)
Seborrhea
Urticaria
Xerosis

Hair
Hair – alopecia

Cardiovascular
Flushing

Other
Anaphylactoid reactions
Galactorrhea (<1%)
Gynecomastia
Hypertrophic papillae of tongue
Mastodynia (1–10%)
Paresthesias
Priapism (<1%)
Sialorrhea
Tremor
Xerostomia

METHADONE

Trade name: Dolphine (Roxane)
Other common trade names: *Eptadone; L-Polamidon; Mephenon; Metadon; Methadose; Physeptone*
Indications: Pain, narcotic addiction
Category: Antitussive; Narcotic analgesic; Suppressant (narcotic abstinence syndrome)
Half-life: 15–25 hours
Clinically important, potentially hazardous interactions with: diazepam, erythromycin, fluconazole, fluvoxamine, **St John's wort**

Reactions

Skin
 Angioedema
 Cellulitis [1]
 Diaphoresis (<48%) [3]
 Exanthems
 Facial edema
 Pruritus (<1%)
 Purpura
 Rash (sic) (<1%)
 Urticaria (<1%)

Cardiovascular
 Flushing

QT prolongation [1]
Torsades de pointes [5]

Other
 Death [8]
 Headache
 Injection-site burning
 Injection-site induration
 Injection-site pain (1–10%)
 Rhabdomyolysis [1]
 Tremor [1]
 Xerostomia (1–10%)

METHAMPHETAMINE

Trade name: Desoxyn (Ovation)
Indications: Attention deficit disorder, obesity
Category: Central nervous system stimulant; Recreational drug
Half-life: 4–5 hours
Clinically important, potentially hazardous interactions with: fluoxetine, fluvoxamine, MAO inhibitors, paroxetine, phenelzine, sertraline, tranylcypromine

Reactions

Skin
 Acaraphobia [1]
 Diaphoresis (1–10%)
 Lichenoid eruption [1]
 Nodular eruption [1]
 Pigmentation [1]
 Rash (sic) (<1%)

Toxic epidermal necrolysis [1]
Urticaria (<1%)

Cardiovascular
 Angina [1]

Other
 Anxiety [1]
 Death [2]

Delusions of parasitosis [1]
Depression [1]
Dysgeusia
Gynecomastia [1]
Headache

Injection-site lipoatrophy [1]
Polyarteritis nodosa [2]
Rhabdomyolysis (43%) [5]
Tremor
Xerostomia (1–10%)

METHOHEXITAL

Trade name: Brevital
Other common trade names: *Brevimytal; Brietal; Brietal Sodium*
Indications: General anesthesia
Category: Barbiturate; General anesthetic
Half-life: 4–8 minutes

Reactions

Skin
 Angioedema [2]
 Erythema
 Exanthems [1]
 Rash (sic)
 Urticaria [2]

Other
 Anaphylactoid reactions

Injection-site edema
Injection-site pain (18%)
Injection-site phlebitis [1]
Rhabdomyolysis [1]
Sialorrhea
Thrombophlebitis (<1%)
Tremor

METHSUXIMIDE

Trade name: Celontin (Pfizer)
Other common trade name: *Petinutin*
Indications: Absence (petit-mal) seizures
Category: Succinimide anticonvulsant
Half-life: 2–4 hours

Reactions

Skin
 Acanthosis nigricans [1]
 Erythema multiforme
 Exanthems [1]
 Exfoliative dermatitis (<1%)
 Lupus erythematosus (>10%)
 Pruritus
 Purpura
 Rash (sic)
 Stevens–Johnson syndrome (>10%)
 Urticaria (<1%)

Hair
 Hair – alopecia
 Hair – hirsutism

Eyes
 Periorbital edema

Other
 Gingival hypertrophy
 Headache
 Oral ulceration

METOCLOPRAMIDE

Trade name: Reglan (Wyeth)
Other common trade names: *Apo-Metoclop; Duraclamid; Emex; Gastrocil; Gastronerton; Maxeran; Maxolon; Mygdalon; Primperan*
Indications: Gastroesophageal reflux
Category: Antiemetic; Dopaminergic blocking agent; Peristaltic stimulant
Half-life: 4–6 hours
Clinically important, potentially hazardous interactions with: mepenzolate, sertraline, venlafaxine

Reactions

Skin
  Allergic reactions (sic) [1]
  Angioedema [2]
  Diaphoresis [1]
  Exanthems [3]
  Rash (sic) (1–10%)
  Urticaria [2]

Cardiovascular
  Flushing

Other
  Dyskinesia [1]

  Galactorrhea
  Gynecomastia [1]
  Mastodynia (1–10%)
  Paresthesias [1]
  Parkinsonism [2]
  Porphyria [2]
  Serotonin syndrome [2]
  Tardive dyskinesia [1]
  Tongue pigmentation [1]
  Xerostomia (1–10%)

MIDAZOLAM

Trade name: Versed (Roche)
Other common trade name: *Dormicum*
Indications: Preoperative sedation
Category: Anesthetic; Benzodiazepine sedative-analgesic; Benzodiazepine sedative-hypnotic
Half-life: 1–4 hours
Clinically important, potentially hazardous interactions with: amprenavir, aprepitant, atazanavir, carbamazepine, chlorpheniramine, cimetidine, clarithromycin, clorazepate, CNS depressants, delavirdine, dexamethasone, efavirenz, erythromycin, esomeprazole, fluconazole, fluoxetine, fosamprenavir, **grapefruit juice**, griseofulvin, imatinib, indinavir, itraconazole, ivermectin, ketoconazole, nelfinavir, nevirapine, phenobarbital, phenytoin, primidone, rifabutin, rifampin, ritonavir, saquinavir, **St John's wort**, telithromycin

Reactions

Skin
  Adverse effects [1]
  Angioedema [1]

  Exanthems
  Peripheral edema (<1%)
  Pruritus (<1%) [1]

Rash (sic) (<1%)
Urticaria (<1%)

Cardiovascular
Hypotension [1]

Other
Anaphylactoid reactions (<1%)

Dysgeusia (<1%) (acid taste)
Headache
Injection-site pain (>10%) [1]
Injection-site reactions (sic) (>10%)
Paresthesias
Sialorrhea (<1%)

MIRTAZAPINE

Trade name: Remeron (Organon)
Indications: Depression
Category: Alpha-2-adrenoceptor blocker; Tetracyclic antidepressant
Half-life: 20–40 hours
Clinically important, potentially hazardous interactions with: telithromycin

Reactions

Skin
Acne
Allergic reactions (sic) [1]
Cellulitis
Chills
Diaphoresis [1]
Edema (1–10%) [1]
Exfoliative dermatitis
Facial edema
Flu-like syndrome (1–10%) [1]
Herpes simplex
Peripheral edema (1–10%) [1]
Petechiae
Photosensitivity
Pruritus
Rash (sic) (1–10%) [1]
Seborrhea
Ulcerations
Xerosis

Other
Ageusia
Anxiety [1]
Aphthous stomatitis
Arthralgia [2]

Dysgeusia
Fatigue [2]
Glossitis (1–10%)
Gynecomastia
Headache [1]
Hyperesthesia
Mastodynia
Myalgia (1–10%) [1]
Oral candidiasis
Paresthesias [1]
Parosmia
Phlebitis
Restless legs syndrome [3]
Rhabdomyolysis [1]
Serotonin syndrome [4]
Sialorrhea
Stomatitis
Tendon rupture
Tongue edema
Tongue pigmentation
Tremor (1–10%) [1]
Vaginitis
Xerostomia (25%) [1]

MISTLETOE

Scientific names: *Phoradendron flavescens; Phoradendron leucarpum; Phoradendron macrophyllum; Phoradendron rubrum; Phoradendron serotinum; Phoradendron tomentosum; Viscum album*
Family: Loranthacae; Viscaceae
Trade and other common names: ABNOBA viscum; All-heal; Devil's fuge; Eurixor; Folia Visci; Helixor; Herbe de la Croix; Iscador (Weleda); Isorel (Novipharm); Lektinol; Lignum Crucis; Stipites Visci; VaQuFrF (Labor Hiscia); Vysorel
Category: Adjuvant; Immune modulator
Purported indications and other uses: Injected: adjuvant tumor therapy. **Oral:** abortifacient, arteriosclerosis, arthritis, asthma, colds, depression, headache, HIV infection, hypertension, hypotension, hysteria, labor pain, lumbago, metrorrhagia, muscle spasms, otitis, whooping cough, hemorrhoids, internal bleeding, gout, sleep disorders, amenorrhea, liver and gallbladder conditions
Half-life: N/A
Clinically important, potentially hazardous interactions with: bepridil, corticosteroids, digoxin, diltiazem, immunosuppressants, MAO inhibitors, verapamil

Note: Purified extracts injected intramuscularly, subcutaneously or by intravenous infusion. Unless otherwise indicated, side effects listed are from injected preparations. The FDA considers *Viscum album* unsafe

Reactions

Skin
   Adverse effects (sic) [2]
   Allergic reactions (sic) [3]
   Chills [2]
   Dermatitis [1]
   Edema of lip [1]
   Erythema [3]
   Flu-like syndrome [2]
   Nodular eruption [1]
   Pruritus [1]
Other
   Anaphylactoid reactions (28%) [2]
   Death (low incidence – accidental ingestion) [4]
   Gingivitis [2]
   Injection-site edema [1]
   Injection-site inflammation [6]

*Note: The well-known mistletoe is an evergreen parasitic plant, growing on the branches of some tree species

**Note: Shakespeare calls it 'the baleful mistletoe,' an illusion to the Scandinavian legend that Balder, the god of Peace, was slain with an arrow made of mistletoe

MOLINDONE

Trade name: Moban (Endo)
Indications: Schizophrenia
Category: Antipsychotic
Half-life: 1.5 hours

Reactions

Skin
 Allergic reactions (sic)
 Edema
 Hypohidrosis (<1%)
 Peripheral edema
 Photosensitivity (<1%)
 Pigmentation (<1%)
 Pruritus (<1%)

Rash (sic) (<1%)

Other
 Galactorrhea (<1%)
 Gynecomastia (1–10%)
 Sialorrhea
 Xerostomia (>10%)

MORPHINE

Trade names: Astramorph; Avinza (Ligand); Duramorph (Baxter) (Elkins-Sinn); Infumorph (Baxter); Kadian (aaiPharma); MS Contin (Purdue); MS/S; MSIR Oral (Purdue); OMS Oral; Oramorph SR; RMS; Roxanol (aaiPharma)
Other common trade names: *Anamorph; Astramorph; Contalgin; Epimorph; Morphine-HP; MOS; Moscontin; MS-IR; MST Continus; Sevredol; Statex*
Indications: Severe pain, acute myocardial infarction
Category: Narcotic analgesic
Half-life: 2–4 hours
Clinically important, potentially hazardous interactions with: buprenorphine*, cimetidine, furazolidone, MAO inhibitors, pentazocine

Reactions

Skin
 Diaphoresis [1]
 Edema
 Exanthems [1]
 Pallor
 Peripheral edema
 Pruritus (5–65%) [17]
 Pustular psoriasis [1]
 Rash (sic)

Cardiovascular
 Bradycardia [1]
 Flushing

Hypotension [1]

Other
 Death [1]
 Gynecomastia
 Hyperalgesia [1]
 Hyperesthesia
 Injection-site pain (>10%)
 Rhabdomyolysis [2]
 Trembling (1–10%)
 Xerostomia (>10%) [2]

NALBUPHINE

Trade name: Nubain (Endo)
Other common trade names: *Bufigen; Nalcryn SP; Nubain SP*
Indications: Moderate to severe pain
Category: Narcotic agonist-antagonistic analgesic
Half-life: 5 hours
Clinically important, potentially hazardous interactions with: CNS depressants, diazepam, pentobarbital, promethazine

Note: Nalbuphine contains sulfites

Reactions

Skin
Burning (<1%) [1]
Clammy skin (9%)
Diaphoresis (9%)
Pruritus (<1%)
Urticaria (<1%)

Eyes
Blurred vision

Cardiovascular
Flushing (<1%)

Other
Depression (<1%)
Dizziness (5%) [1]
Dysgeusia (<1%)
Headache
Injection-site pain [2]
Numbness
Paresthesias
Tingling
Xerostomia (4%)

NALOXONE

Trade names: Narcan (Endo); Suboxone (Reckitt Benckiser); Talwin-NX (Sanofi-Aventis)
Other common trade names: *Nalpin; Narcanti; Narcotan; Zynox*
Indications: Narcotic overdose
Category: Opioid (narcotic) antagonist
Half-life: 1–1.5 hours

Reactions

Skin
Angioedema [1]
Diaphoresis (1–10%)
Exanthems
Pruritus [1]
Rash (sic) (1–10%)

Urticaria [1]

Other
Headache
Hyperalgesia [1]

NALTREXONE

Trade names: Revex (Baxter); ReVia (Meda); Trexan
Other common trade names: *Antaxone; Celupan; Nalorex; Nemexin*
Indications: Substance abuse, opioid dependence, alcohol dependence
Category: Opioid antagonist
Half-life: 4 hours

Reactions

Skin
  Acne (<1%)
  Chills (<10%)
  Diaphoresis
  Edema (<1%)
  Exanthems [1]
  Herpes simplex (<1%)
  Herpes zoster (<1%)
  Pruritus (<1%) [2]
  Purpura
  Rash (sic) (<10%) [1]
  Seborrhea (<1%)
  Tinea (<1%)

Hair
  Hair – alopecia (<1%)

Eyes
  Eyelid edema (<1%)

Cardiovascular
  Hot flashes

Other
  Arthralgia (>10%) [1]
  Death (in ultrarapid detoxification)
  Depression (<1%) [2]
  Myalgia
  Phlebitis (<1%)
  Rhabdomyolysis [1]
  Tinnitus
  Tremor
  Twitching
  Xerostomia (<1%)

NARATRIPTAN

Trade name: Amerge (GSK)
Indications: Acute migraine attacks
Category: Antimigraine; Serotonin agonist
Half-life: 6 hours
Clinically important, potentially hazardous interactions with: dihydroergotamine, ergotamine, methysergide, rizatriptan, sibutramine, **St John's wort**, sumatriptan, zolmitriptan

Reactions

Skin
  Acne (<1%)
  Allergic reactions (sic) (<1%)
  Dermatitis (<1%)
  Diaphoresis (<1%)
  Edema (<1%)
  Erythema (<1%)
  Exanthems (<1%)
  Folliculitis (<1%)
  Photosensitivity (<1%)
  Purpura (<1%)
  Rash (sic) (<1%)
  Sensitivity (sic) (<1)%
  Urticaria (<1%)

Xerosis (<1%)

Hair

Hair – alopecia (<1%)

Eyes

Ocular pigmentation (<1%)

Other

Dysgeusia (<1%)
Headache
Hyperesthesia (<1%)
Paresthesias (2%)
Sialopenia (<1%)

NEFAZODONE

Trade name: Serzone (Bristol-Myers Squibb)
Indications: Depression
Category: Phenylpiperazine antidepressant
Half-life: 2–4 hours
Clinically important, potentially hazardous interactions with: aprepitant, buspirone, isocarboxazid, MAO inhibitors, phenelzine, pimozide, selegiline, sibutramine, solifenacin, **St John's wort**, sumatriptan, telithromycin, tramadol, tranylcypromine, trazodone

Reactions

Skin

Acne (<1%)
Allergic reactions (sic) (<1%)
Burning [1]
Cellulitis (<1%)
Eczema (<1%)
Exanthems (<1%)
Facial edema (<1%)
Flu-like syndrome (1–10%)
Infections (8%)
Peripheral edema (3%)
Photosensitivity (<1%)
Pruritus (2%)
Rash (sic) (2%)
Urticaria (<1%)
Vesiculobullous eruption (<1%)
Xerosis (<1%)

Hair

Hair – alopecia (<1%) [2]

Hematopoietic

Ecchymoses (<1%)

Cardiovascular

Flushing (4%)

Other

Ageusia (<1%)
Death [1]
Dysgeusia (2%)
Foetor ex ore (halitosis) (<1%)
Gingivitis (<1%)
Glossitis (<1%)
Gynecomastia (<1%)
Headache
Hyperesthesia (<1%)
Mastodynia (1%)
Myalgia
Oral candidiasis (<1%)
Oral ulceration (<1%)
Paresthesias (4%) [1]
Priapism (<1%) [1]
Rhabdomyolysis [2]
Sialorrhea (<1%)
Stomatitis (<1%)
Vaginitis (2%)
Xerostomia (25%)

NORTRIPTYLINE

Trade names: Aventyl (Ranbaxy); Pamelor (Mallinckrodt)
Other common trade names: *Allegron; Apo-Nortriptyline; Noritren; Norpress; Nortrilen; Paxtibi; Vividyl*
Indications: Depression
Category: Tricyclic antidepressant
Half-life: 28–31 hours
Clinically important, potentially hazardous interactions with: amprenavir, arbutamine, clonidine, epinephrine, fluoxetine, formoterol, guanethidine, isocarboxazid, linezolid, MAO inhibitors, phenelzine, quinolones, sparfloxacin, tranylcypromine

---

Reactions

Skin

Acne
Allergic reactions (sic) (<1%)
Diaphoresis (1–10%)
Edema
Erythema
Exanthems
Petechiae
Photosensitivity (<1%) [2]
Phototoxicity
Pruritus
Purpura
Rash (sic)
Urticaria
Vasculitis
Xerosis

Hair

Hair – alopecia (<1%)

Cardiovascular

Flushing
QT prolongation [1]

Other

Acute intermittent porphyria [1]
Black tongue [1]
Dizziness [1]
Dysgeusia (>10%)
Galactorrhea (<1%)
Gynecomastia (<1%)
Paresthesias
Parkinsonism (1–10%)
Stomatitis
Tinnitus
Tongue edema
Tremor
Vaginitis
Xerostomia (>10%) [2]

OLANZAPINE

Synonym: LY170053
Trade name: Zyprexa (Lilly)
Indications: Psychotic disorders
Category: Benzodiazepine antipsychotic
Half-life: 21–54 hours

Reactions

Skin

Angioedema [1]
Candidiasis (<1%)
Dermatitis (<1%)
Diaphoresis (>1%)
Eczema (<1%)
Edema
Exanthems (<1%)
Facial edema (<1%)
Neuroleptic malignant syndrome [12]
Peripheral edema (3%) [2]
Photosensitivity (<1%)
Pigmentation (<1%) [1]
Pruritus (>1%)
Pustules [1]
Rash (sic) (>2%) [2]
Seborrhea (<1%)
Ulcerations (<1%)
Urticaria (<1%)
Vesiculobullous eruption (2%)
Xanthomas [1]
Xerosis (<1%)

Hair

Hair – alopecia (<1%) [2]
Hair – hirsutism (<1%)

Hematopoietic

Ecchymoses (>1%)

Cardiovascular

Coronary artery disorders [1]
QT prolongation [1]

Other

Akathisia [3]
Aphthous stomatitis (<1%)
Death [1]
Diabetes mellitus [1]
Dizziness [1]
Dysgeusia (<1%)
Fever [1]
Galactorrhea [1]
Gingivitis (<1%)
Glossitis (<1%)
Headache [1]
Hyperesthesia (<1%)
Hypersensitivity [1]
Myalgia (>1%) [1]
Oral candidiasis (<1%)
Oral ulceration (<1%)
Parkinsonism (1–10%) [1]
Priapism (<1%) [9]
Rhabdomyolysis [4]
Seizures [2]
Serotonin syndrome [1]
Sialorrhea (<1%) [1]
Stomatitis (<1%)
Tardive dyskinesia [3]
Tongue edema (<1%) [1]
Tongue pigmentation (<1%)
Tremor (1–10%) [2]
Twitching (2%)
Vaginitis (>1%)
Xerostomia (13%) [5]

ONDANSETRON

Trade name: Zofran (GSK)
Other common trade names: *Emeset; Oncoden; Zofron*
Indications: Nausea and vomiting
Category: Antiemetic; Serotonin antagonist
Half-life: 4 hours
Clinically important, potentially hazardous interactions with: eucalyptus

Reactions

Skin
 Angioedema
 Chills (5–10%)
 Exanthems
 Fixed eruption [2]
 Pruritus (5%)
 Rash (sic) (<1%)
 Urticaria

Hair
 Hair – alopecia

Cardiovascular
 Flushing [1]
 QT prolongation [1]

Other
 Anaphylactoid reactions [3]
 Dysgeusia [1]
 Headache
 Hypersensitivity (<1%) [1]
 Injection-site burning
 Injection-site erythema
 Injection-site pain
 Injection-site reactions (sic) (4%)
 Paresthesias (2%)
 Porphyria [1]
 Sialopenia (1–5%)
 Xerostomia (1–10%) [2]

OXAZEPAM

Trade name: Serax (Mayne)
Other common trade names: *Adumbran; Apo-Oxazepam; Azutranquil; Durazepam; Murelax; Novoxapam; Oxpam; Praxiten; Serax; Serepax; Zapex*
Indications: Anxiety, depression
Category: Anticonvulsant; Benzodiazepine sedative-hypnotic
Half-life: 3–6 hours
Clinically important, potentially hazardous interactions with: amprenavir, chlorpheniramine, clarithromycin, efavirenz, esomeprazole, imatinib, nelfinavir

Reactions

Skin
 Dermatitis (1–10%)
 Diaphoresis (>10%)
 Edema
 Erythema multiforme [1]
 Exanthems

 Fixed eruption [1]
 Pruritus
 Purpura
 Rash (sic) (>10%)
 Toxic epidermal necrolysis [1]
 Urticaria

Other
Headache
Paresthesias
Sialopenia (>10%)

Sialorrhea (1–10%)
Tongue furry
Tremor
Xerostomia (>10%)

OXCARBAZEPINE

Synonym: GP 47680
Trade name: Trileptal (Novartis)
Indications: Partial epileptic seizures
Category: Anticonvulsant
Half-life: 1–2.5 hours

Reactions

Skin
Acne
Allergic reactions (sic) (2%) [2]
Angioedema
Dermatitis
Diaphoresis (3%)
Eczema
Edema (2%)
Erythema multiforme
Exanthems [2]
Facial rash (sic)
Folliculitis
Genital pruritus
Infections (2%)
Lupus erythematosus
Photosensitivity
Purpura (2%)
Rash (sic) (<6%) [1]
Sensitivity [1]
Stevens–Johnson syndrome
Toxic epidermal necrolysis

Vitiligo
Hair
Hair – alopecia
Cardiovascular
Hot flashes (2%)
Other
Dysgeusia (5%)
Gingival hypertrophy
Headache
Hyperesthesia (3%)
Hypersensitivity [1]
Oral ulceration [1]
Priapism
Stomatitis
Toothache (2%)
Tremor (4–6%)
Ulcerative stomatitis
Vaginitis (2%)
Xerostomia (3%)

PALONOSETRON

Trade name: Aloxi (MGI)
Indications: Antiemetic (for cancer chemotherapy)
Category: 5-HT$_3$ receptor antagonist
Half-life: 40 hours

Reactions

Skin
  Dermatitis (<1%)
  Flu-like syndrome (<1%)
  Pruritus (8–22%)
  Rash (sic) (6%)

Cardiovascular
  Hot flashes (<15)

Other
  Anxiety (1%)
  Dizziness (1%)
  Headache (9%)
  Paresthesias
  Xerostomia (<1%)

PARAMETHADIONE

Indications: Absence (petit-mal) seizures
Category: Anticonvulsant
Half-life: 12–24 hours

Reactions

Skin
  Acne
  Erythema multiforme [2]
  Exanthems
  Exfoliative dermatitis [1]
  Lupus erythematosus
  Pruritus

Hair
  Hair – alopecia

Other
  Gingivitis
  Oral mucosal eruption [1]
  Paresthesias

PAROXETINE

Trade name: Paxil (GSK)
Other common trade name: *Aropax 20*
Indications: Depression
Category: Antidepressant; Selective serotonin reuptake inhibitor (SSRI)
Half-life: 21 hours
Clinically important, potentially hazardous interactions with: amphetamines, aprepitant, clarithromycin, dextroamphetamine, diethylpropion, duloxetine, erythromycin, isocarboxazid, linezolid, MAO inhibitors, mazindol, methamphetamine, phendimetrazine, phenelzine, phentermine, phenylpropanolamine, pseudoephedrine, risperidone, selegiline, sibutramine, **St John's wort**, sumatriptan, sympathomimetics, tranylcypromine, trazodone, troleandomycin

Reactions

Skin
  Acne (<1%)
  Allergic reactions (sic) (<1%) [1]
  Angioedema (<1%) [1]

Candidiasis
Dermatitis (<1%)
Diaphoresis (11.2%) [7]
Eczema

Edema (<1%)
Erythema multiforme [1]
Erythema nodosum (<1%)
Exanthems (<1%)
Facial edema (<1%)
Furunculosis (<1%)
Melanoma (<1%)
Neuroleptic malignant syndrome [1]
Peripheral edema (<1%)
Photosensitivity (<1%) [2]
Pigmentation (<1%)
Pruritus (<1%) [1]
Psoriasis [1]
Purpura (<1%)
Rash (sic) (1.7%)
Toxic epidermal necrolysis [1]
Urticaria (<1%)
Vasculitis [1]
Xerosis (<1%)

Hair
Hair – alopecia (<1%) [1]

Hematopoietic
Ecchymoses (<1%) [1]

Cardiovascular
Flushing [1]
QT prolongation [1]

Other
Ageusia (<1%) [1]
Anosmia [1]
Aphthous stomatitis (<1%)
Bruxism (<1%) [1]
Cough [1]
Death [1]
Depression [1]
Dysgeusia (2.4%) [1]
Galactorrhea [2]
Gingivitis (<1%)
Glossitis (<1%)
Headache [1]
Lymphedema
Myalgia (1–10%)
Oral ulceration
Paresthesias (3.8%)
Priapism [1]
Serotonin syndrome [1]
Sialorrhea (<1%)
Stomatitis (<1%)
Tinnitus
Tongue edema (<1%) [1]
Tremor (1–10%)
Vaginitis
Vulvovaginal candidiasis (<1%)
Xerostomia (18.1%) [10]

PEMOLINE

Trade name: Cylert (Abbott)
Other common trade names: *Betanamin; Tradon*
Indications: Attention deficit disorder, narcolepsy
Category: Anorexiant; Central nervous system stimulant
Half-life: 9–14 hours
Clinically important, potentially hazardous interactions with: pimozide

Reactions

Skin
Exanthems (<1%) [1]
Rash (sic) (>10%)

Other
Headache

Parkinsonism
Rhabdomyolysis [1]
Tourette's syndrome

PENTAZOCINE

Trade name: Talwin (Hospira)
Other common trade names: *Fortral; Fortwin; Liticon; Ospronim; Pentafen; Sosegon; Susevin; Talacen*
Indications: Pain
Category: Narcotic; Opioid analgesic; Sedative
Half-life: 2–3 hours
Clinically important, potentially hazardous interactions with: cimetidine, morphine

Reactions

Skin
Cellulitis [1]
Dermatitis
Diaphoresis
Exanthems [1]
Facial edema
Generalized eruption (sic) [1]
Pigmentation (surrounding ulcers) [1]
Pruritus (<1%)
Rash (sic) (1–10%)
Scleroderma [2]
Sclerosis [3]
Toxic epidermal necrolysis (<1%) [2]
Ulcerations [6]
Urticaria

Cardiovascular
Flushing [1]

Other
Dysgeusia
Embolia cutis medicamentosa (Nicolau syndrome) [1]
Fibromyalgia [2]
Injection-site calcification [2]
Injection-site fibrosis [1]
Injection-site granuloma [3]
Injection-site induration [9]
Injection-site pain
Injection-site pigmentation [1]
Lipogranulomas [1]
Myofibrosis [1]
Panniculitis (chronic) [1]
Paresthesias
Phlebitis [1]
Soft tissue calcification [1]
Tinnitus
Xerostomia (1–10%)

PENTOBARBITAL

Other common trade names: *Medinox Mono; Mintal; Nova Rectal; Pentobarbitone; Prodromol; Sombutol*

Indications: Insomnia, sedation

Category: Anticonvulsant; Barbiturate sedative-hypnotic

Half-life: 15–50 hours

Clinically important, potentially hazardous interactions with: alcohol, anticoagulants, antihistamines, brompheniramine, buclizine, chlorpheniramine, dicumarol, ethanolamine, imatinib, nalbuphine, warfarin

Reactions

Skin
  Acne
  Angioedema (<1%)
  Bullous eruption [1]
  Erythema multiforme [1]
  Exanthems [1]
  Exfoliative dermatitis (<1%) [1]
  Fixed eruption [1]
  Herpes simplex (activation)
  Lupus erythematosus [2]
  Necrosis [1]
  Photosensitivity [1]
  Pruritus
  Purpura [1]
  Rash (sic) (<1%)

  Stevens–Johnson syndrome (<1%)
  Toxic epidermal necrolysis [1]
  Urticaria
  Vasculitis

Other
  Headache
  Hypersensitivity
  Injection-site pain (1–10%)
  Injection-site reactions (sic) (<1%)
  Oral ulceration
  Porphyria [1]
  Porphyria variegata
  Rhabdomyolysis [1]
  Thrombophlebitis (<1%)

PEPPERMINT

Scientific name: *Mentha piperita*

Family: Labiatae

Trade and other common names: Aludrox; brandy mint; Colpermin; Enteroplant (peppermint and caraway oils); menthol; PCC

Category: Analgesic; Antemetic; Antiseptic; Carminative; Cholagogue; Choleretic; Diaphoretic; Disinfectant; Peripheral vasodilator; Spasmolytic

Purported indications and other uses: Dyspepsia, regress pancreatic, mammary, and liver tumors, irritable bowel syndrome, colonic spasm, colic, nausea, vomiting, biliary disorders, common cold, dysmenorrhoea, anxiolytic. **Topical:** pain, itching, inflammations, headaches, toothache, pruritus, urticaria, mosquito repellant. Vapor: bronchial catarrh, fever, influenza. Flavoring, cosmetics, toothpaste, mouthwash

Half-life: N/A

Clinically important, potentially hazardous interactions with: cisapride

Reactions

Skin
Adverse effects (sic) [2]
Allergic reactions (sic) [1]
Burning (anal) [1]
Cheilitis [2]
Dermatitis [3]
Lichenoid eruption [1]
Perioral dermatitis [1]
Rash (sic) [1]
Sensitivity [2]

Other
Burning mouth syndrome [1]
Gingivitis [1]
Glossitis [1]
Hypersensitivity [2]
Oral ulceration [2]
Side effects (sic) [2]
Stomatitis [2]
Toxicity [1]

PERPHENAZINE

Trade names: Etrafon; Trilafon (Schering)
Other common trade names: *Apo-Perphenzine; Decentan; Fentazin; Leptopsique; Peratsin; Perphenan; Trilifan Retard; Triomin*
Indications: Psychotic disorders, nausea and vomiting
Category: Phenothiazine antipsychotic
Half-life: 9 hours
Clinically important, potentially hazardous interactions with: sparfloxacin

Etrafon and Triavil are combinations of perphenazine and amitriptyline

Reactions

Skin
Angioedema
Dermatitis
Diaphoresis
Eczema
Erythema
Exanthems [2]
Exfoliative dermatitis
Lupus erythematosus [4]
Peripheral edema
Photosensitivity
Pigmentation (blue-gray) (<1%)
Pruritus
Purpura
Rash (sic) (1–10%)
Seborrhea
Urticaria [1]
Xerosis

Cardiovascular
Congestive heart failure [1]

Other
Anaphylactoid reactions
Galactorrhea (black) (<1%) [1]
Gynecomastia
Headache
Mastodynia (1–10%)
Parkinsonism
Priapism (<1%)
Pseudolymphoma [1]
Rhabdomyolysis [1]
Sialorrhea
Tardive dyskinesia [1]
Tinnitus
Xerostomia

PHENDIMETRAZINE

Trade name: Bontril (Amarin)
Other common trade name: *Obesan-X*
Indications: Obesity
Category: Appetite suppressant
Half-life: 5–12.5 hours
Clinically important, potentially hazardous interactions with: fluoxetine, fluvoxamine, MAO inhibitors, paroxetine, phenelzine, sertraline, tranylcypromine

Reactions

Skin
  Diaphoresis
  Urticaria

Cardiovascular
  Flushing

Other
  Dysgeusia
  Headache
  Xerostomia

PHENELZINE

Trade name: Nardil (Pfizer)
Other common trade name: *Nardelzine*
Indications: Depression
Category: Antidepressant; Monoamine oxidase (MAO) inhibitor
Half-life: N/A
Clinically important, potentially hazardous interactions with: amitriptyline, amoxapine, amphetamines, bupropion, citalopram, clomipramine, cyproheptadine, desipramine, dextroamphetamine, dextromethorphan, diethylpropion, dopamine, doxepin, entacapone, **ephedra**, ephedrine, epinephrine, fluoxetine, fluvoxamine, **ginseng**, imipramine, levodopa, mazindol, meperidine, methamphetamine, nefazodone, nortriptyline, paroxetine, phendimetrazine, phentermine, phenylephrine, protriptyline, pseudoephedrine, rizatriptan, sertraline, sibutramine, sumatriptan, sympathomimetics, tramadol, tricyclic antidepressants, trimipramine, **tryptophan***, venlafaxine, zolmitriptan

Reactions

Skin
  Angioedema [1]
  Diaphoresis [1]
  Edema
  Exanthems
  Lupus erythematosus [1]
  Peripheral edema [2]
  Photosensitivity [2]

  Pruritus (13%) [1]
  Rash (sic)
  Telangiectasia
  Urticaria

Other
  Black tongue
  Glossitis [1]
  Headache

Parkinsonism
Priapism
Rhabdomyolysis [1]

Tremor
Twitching
Xerostomia (1–10%) [1]

PHENOBARBITAL

Synonyms: phenobarbitone; phenylethylmalonylurea
Trade names: Barbita; Luminal (Sanofi-Aventis); Solfoton
Other common trade names: *Alepsal; Barbilixir; Barbital; Gardenal; Luminaletten; Phenaemal; Phenobarbitone*
Indications: Insomnia, seizures
Category: Barbiturate sedative-hypnotic
Half-life: 2–6 days
Clinically important, potentially hazardous interactions with: alcohol, anticoagulants, antihistamines, brompheniramine, buclizine, chlorpheniramine, delavirdine, dicumarol, ethanolamine, fluconazole, fosamprenavir, imatinib, **influenza vaccines**, meperidine, midazolam, solifenacin, telithromycin, warfarin

Reactions

Skin
Acne [1]
Acute generalized exanthematous
  pustulosis (AGEP) [1]
Allergic reactions (sic) [2]
Angioedema (<1%)
Anticonvulsant hypersensitivity syndrome
  [3]
Bullous eruption [5]
Depigmentation [1]
Edema
Erythema multiforme [7]
Erythroderma [1]
Exanthems [10]
Exfoliative dermatitis (<1%) [6]
Fixed eruption [7]
Graft-versus-host reaction [1]
Herpes simplex (activation)
Lupus erythematosus [2]
Necrosis [1]
Pemphigus [1]
Peripheral edema [1]
Photosensitivity [1]
Pruritus [1]

Purpura [2]
Pustules (generalized) [1]
Rash (sic) (<1%)
Stevens–Johnson syndrome (<1%) [12]
Toxic epidermal necrolysis [19]
Toxicoderma [1]
Urticaria [1]
Vasculitis

Hair
Hair – depigmentation [1]

Nails
Nails – hypoplasia [2]

Other
Acute intermittent porphyria [1]
Death
DRESS syndrome [4]
Gingival hypertrophy [1]
Headache
Hypersensitivity (<1%)* [7]
Hypoplasia of phalanges [2]
Injection-site bullous eruption [1]
Injection-site pain (>10%)
Injection-site thrombophlebitis (>10%)

Oral ulceration
Osteomalacia [1]
Porphyria cutanea tarda [1]

Porphyria variegata
Rhabdomyolysis [1]
Xerostomia [1]

PHENSUXIMIDE

Indications: Petit mal seizures
Category: Anticonvulsant
Half-life: 5–12 hours

Reactions

Skin
Erythema multiforme (<1%)
Lupus erythematosus
Pruritus
Purpura [1]
Rash (sic)
Stevens–Johnson syndrome

Hair
Hair – alopecia

Hair – hirsutism

Eyes
Periorbital edema

Other
Acute intermittent porphyria
Gingival hypertrophy
Oral ulceration

PHENTERMINE

Trade names: Adipex-P (Gate); Ionamin (Celltech)
Other common trade names: *Behapront; Diminex; Minobese-Forte; Panbesy; Panbesyl; Redusa; Umine; Zantryl*
Indications: Obesity
Category: Appetite suppressant (anorexiant)
Half-life: 19–24 hours
Clinically important, potentially hazardous interactions with: fluoxetine, fluvoxamine, MAO inhibitors, paroxetine, phenelzine, sertraline, tranylcypromine

Reactions

Skin
Diaphoresis (<1%)
Peripheral edema
Peripheral vasculopathy [1]
Purpura
Rash (sic)
Raynaud's phenomenon [1]
Urticaria

Hair
Hair – alopecia (<1%)

Cardiovascular
QT prolongation [1]

Other
Dysgeusia
Headache
Myalgia (<1%)
Tremor
Xerostomia

PHENYLPROPANOLAMINE

Synonym: PPA
Trade names: Acutrim; BC Cold Powder; Control; Dex-a-Diet; Dexatrim; Diet Gum; Genex; Maigret-50; Phenoxine; Phenyldrine; Prolamine; Propagest; Propandrine; Rhindecon; Spray-U-Thin; St. Joseph Aspirin-Free Cold Tablets (McNeil); Stay Trim; Unitrol; Westrim
Indications: Nasal decongestion, anorexiant
Category: Adrenergic agonist; Anorexiant; Nasal decongestant; Sympathomimetic
Half-life: 3–4 hours
Clinically important, potentially hazardous interactions with: caffeine, ephedra, ephedrine, fluoxetine, fluvoxamine, furazolidone, **guarana,** paroxetine, sertraline, tranylcypromine

Reactions

Skin
  Fixed eruption [1]
  Pallor

Cardiovascular
  QT prolongation [1]

Other
  Death [2]
  Depression
  Rhabdomyolysis [4]
  Tremor
  Xerostomia

PHENYTOIN

Synonyms: diphenylhydantoin; DPH; phenytoin sodium
Trade names: Dilantin (Pfizer); Phenytek (Mylan Bertek)
Other common trade names: *Di-Hydran; Diphenylan; Epanutin; Fenytoin; Phenhydan; Pyoredol; Zentropil*
Indications: Grand mal seizures
Category: Antiarrhythmic; Hydantoin anticonvulsant
Half-life: 7–42 hours (dose dependent)
Clinically important, potentially hazardous interactions with: amprenavir, aprepitant, calcium, chloramphenicol, cimetidine, clorazepate, cyclosporine, delavirdine, diazoxide, disulfiram, dopamine, fluconazole, fluoxetine, fosamprenavir, **ginkgo biloba,** imatinib, indinavir, **influenza vaccines,** isoniazid, isradipine, itraconazole, meperidine, midazolam, nelfinavir, **primrose,** ritonavir, **sage,** saquinavir, solifenacin, **St John's wort,** sucralfate, telithromycin, ticlopidine, vigabatrin

An excellent overview of cutaneous reactions to phenytoin can be found in (1988): Silverman AK+, *J Am Acad Dermatol* 18, 721

Note: About 19% of patients receiving phenytoin develop skin reactions (1983): Rapp RP+, *Neurosurg* 13, 272. They typically develop 10 to 14 days following the start of treatment

Reactions

Skin

Acne [7]
Acute generalized exanthematous
  pustulosis (AGEP) [2]
Angioedema [2]
Anticonvulsant hypersensitivity syndrome
  [2]
Bullous eruption [1]
Dermatomyositis [1]
Eosinophilic fasciitis [1]
Epidermolysis bullosa [1]
Erythema multiforme [11]
Erythroderma [4]
Exanthems (6–71%) [15]
Exfoliative dermatitis [12]
Fixed eruption [3]
Heel pad thickening [1]
Lichen planus [1]
Lichenoid eruption [1]
Linear IgA dermatosis [5]
Lupus erythematosus [16]
Lymphoma (<1%) [5]
Mucocutaneous lymph node syndrome
  (Kawasaki syndrome) [1]
Mycosis fungoides [4]
Necrosis [1]
Pemphigus [1]
Peripheral edema [1]
Pigmentation [1]
Pruritus [6]
Pseudoacanthosis nigricans [1]
Purple glove syndrome [5]
Purpura [4]
Pustules [3]
Rash (sic) (1–10%) [3]
Reticular hyperplasia [2]
Rhinophyma [1]
Scleroderma [1]
Sezary syndrome [1]
Sjøgren's syndrome [1]
Stevens–Johnson syndrome (14%) [27]
Toxic dermatitis [1]

Toxic epidermal necrolysis (2%) [39]
Urticaria [4]
Vasculitis (2%) [6]
Warts [1]

Hair

Hair – alopecia [3]
Hair – hirsutism [5]
Hair – hypertrichosis [2]

Nails

Nails – changes (sic) [2]
Nails – hypoplasia [3]
Nails – onychopathy [1]
Nails – pigmentation [1]

Cardiovascular

Arrhythmias [1]
Bradycardia [1]
Congestive heart failure [1]

Other

Acromegaloid features [1]
Acute intermittent porphyria [1]
Ageusia [2]
Application-site pain [1]
Coarse facies [2]
Death
Digital malformations [3]
Dyskinesia [2]
Fetal hydantoin syndrome* [7]
Gingival hypertrophy (>10%) [27]
Gynecomastia [1]
Headache
Hypersensitivity** [32]
Injection-site extravasation [1]
Injection-site necrosis [2]
Injection-site pain [1]
Lymphadenopathy [1]
Lymphoproliferative disease [1]
Mucocutaneous eruption [2]
Myalgia [2]
Oral ulceration [1]
Osteomalacia [1]
Paresthesias (<1%) [2]

Periarteritis nodosa [2]	Porphyria cutanea tarda [1]
Peyronie's disease	Pseudolymphoma (<1%) [29]
Polyfibromatosis [1]	Rhabdomyolysis [2]
Polymyositis [1]	Serum sickness [2]
Porphyria [1]	Thrombophlebitis (<1%)

*Note: The fetal hydantoin syndrome (FHS) – children whose mothers receive phenytoin during pregnancy are born with FHS. The main features of this syndrome are mental and growth retardation, unusual facies, digital and nail hypoplasia, and coarse scalp hair. Occasionally neonatal acne will be present

PIMOZIDE

Trade name: Orap (Gate)
Other common trade names: *Frenal; Neurap; Pimodac*
Indications: Tourette's syndrome, schizophrenia
Category: Antipsychotic-antidyskinetic (Tourette's syndrome); Neuroleptic agent
Half-life: 50 hours
Clinically important, potentially hazardous interactions with: amphetamines, aprepitant, atazanavir, azithromycin, azole antifungals, clarithromycin, dirithromycin, erythromycin, fluoxetine, fosamprenavir, **grapefruit juice**, imatinib, indinavir, itraconazole, ketoconazole, methylphenidate, nefazodone, nelfinavir, pemoline, phenothiazines, protease inhibitors, quinidine, ritonavir, saquinavir, sertraline, sparfloxacin, telithromycin, thioridazine, tricyclic antidepressants, troleandomycin, voriconazole, zileuton, ziprasidone

Reactions

Skin
  Diaphoresis
  Exanthems
  Facial edema (1–10%)
  Photosensitivity [1]
  Pigmentation [1]
  Pruritus
  Rash (sic) (8.3%)
  Urticaria

Eyes
  Periorbital edema

Cardiovascular
  Arrhythmias [1]

  Torsades de pointes [1]

Other
  Death [1]
  Dysgeusia
  Galactorrhea
  Gynecomastia (>10%)
  Headache
  Myalgia (2.7%)
  Sialorrhea (13.8%) [1]
  Tardive dyskinesia [1]
  Tremor
  Xerostomia (>10%) [3]

PRAZEPAM

Other common trade names: *Centrac; Demetrin; Lysanxia; Prazene; Sedapran; Trepidan*
Indications: Anxiety, depression
Category: Antidepressant; Anxiolytic; Benzodiazepine sedative-hypnotic
Half-life: 30–100 hours

Reactions

Skin
  Dermatitis (1–10%)
  Diaphoresis (>10%)
  Exanthems
  Facial edema
  Peripheral edema
  Pruritus
  Purpura
  Rash (sic) (>10%)
  Urticaria

Hair
  Hair – alopecia
  Hair – hirsutism

Other
  Gingivitis
  Paresthesias
  Sialopenia (>10%)
  Sialorrhea (1–10%)
  Xerostomia (>10%)

PRIMIDONE

Trade name: Mysoline (Xcel)
Other common trade names: *Midone; Mylepsin; PMS Primidone; Prysoline; Sertan*
Indications: Seizures
Category: Anticonvulsant; Barbiturate
Half-life: 10–12 hours
Clinically important, potentially hazardous interactions with: alcohol, anticoagulants, antihistamines, brompheniramine, buclizine, chlorpheniramine, dicumarol, ethanolamine*, imatinib, midazolam, niacinamide, warfarin

Reactions

Skin
  Acne
  Allergic reactions (sic) [1]
  Erythema multiforme (<1%) [3]
  Exanthems (1–5%) [1]
  Exfoliative dermatitis
  Lupus erythematosus (<1%) [6]
  Rash (sic) (<1%)
  Toxic epidermal necrolysis [4]

  Urticaria [1]

Other
  Acute intermittent porphyria
  Gingival hypertrophy
  Hypersensitivity* [2]
  Mucocutaneous syndrome [1]
  Osteomalacia [1]
  Rhabdomyolysis [1]

PROCHLORPERAZINE

Trade name: Compazine (GSK)
Other common trade names: *Edisylate; Novamin; Novomit; Pasotomin; Prorazin; Stella; Stemetil; Tementil; Vertigon*
Indications: Psychotic disorders
Category: Phenothiazine antipsychotic
Half-life: 23 hours
Clinically important, potentially hazardous interactions with: antihistamines, arsenic, chlorpheniramine, dofetilide, piperazine, quinolones, sparfloxacin

Reactions

Skin
  Diaphoresis
  Eczema
  Erythema
  Exanthems [1]
  Exfoliative dermatitis
  Fixed eruption (<1%) [1]
  Hypohidrosis (>10%)
  Lupus erythematosus
  Peripheral edema
  Photosensitivity (1–10%) [3]
  Phototoxicity
  Pigmentation (<1%) (blue-gray)
  Pruritus (1–10%)
  Purpura [1]
  Rash (sic) (1–10%)
  Seborrhea

  Toxic epidermal necrolysis [2]
  Urticaria
  Xerosis

Other
  Anaphylactoid reactions (1–10%)
  Galactorrhea (<1%)
  Gynecomastia (1–10%)
  Headache
  Lip ulceration [1]
  Mastodynia
  Parkinsonism
  Priapism (<1%)
  Sialorrhea
  Tongue pigmentation [1]
  Tremor
  Xerostomia (>10%)

PROMAZINE

Other common trade names: *Liranol; Prazine; Protactyl; Savamine; Talofen*
Indications: Psychotic disorders, schizophrenia
Category: Antiemetic; Phenothiazine antipsychotic
Half-life: 24 hours
Clinically important, potentially hazardous interactions with: sparfloxacin

Reactions

Skin
  Dermatitis
  Edema
  Exanthems [1]

  Hypohidrosis (>10%)
  Photosensitivity (1–10%) [1]
  Phototoxicity [2]
  Pigmentation (<1%) (slate-gray)

Purpura
Rash (sic) (1–10%)
Urticaria
Xerosis

Other
Galactorrhea (<1%)

Gynecomastia
Mastodynia (1–10%)
Parkinsonism
Priapism (<1%)
Xerostomia

PROMETHAZINE

Trade names: Anergan; Phenazine; Phenergan (Wyeth)
Other common trade names: *Atosil; Bonnox; Closin; Goodnight; Histantil; Pentazine; Prometh-50; Prothiazine; Pyrethia*
Indications: Allergic rhinitis, urticaria
Category: Antivertigo; Phenothiazine
Half-life: 10–14 hours
Clinically important, potentially hazardous interactions with: antihistamines, arsenic, chlorpheniramine, dofetilide, nalbuphine, piperazine, quinolones, sparfloxacin

Reactions

Skin
Allergic reactions (sic) (<1%)
Angioedema (<1%)
Bullous eruption (<1%)
Chills
Dermatitis [4]
Diaphoresis
Eczema [1]
Erythema multiforme [2]
Exanthems [1]
Fixed eruption [1]
Jaundice
Lupus erythematosus [2]
Photosensitivity (<1%) [13]
Pigmentation
Purpura [2]
Rash (sic) (<1%) [1]
Stevens–Johnson syndrome [1]
Toxic epidermal necrolysis (<1%) [2]
Urticaria [3]

Cardiovascular
Flushing

Other
Anaphylactoid reactions [1]
Embolia cutis medicamentosa (Nicolau syndrome) [1]
Galactorrhea
Gynecomastia
Headache
Hypersensitivity [1]
Injection-site reactions (sic)
Mastodynia
Myalgia (<1%)
Oral ulceration [1]
Paresthesias (<1%)
Parkinsonism
Priapism
Tinnitus
Xerostomia (1–10%) [1]

PROPOFOL

Trade name: Diprivan (AstraZeneca)
Indications: Induction and maintenance of anesthesia
Category: General anesthetic; Sedative
Half-life: initial: 40 minutes; terminal: 3 days
Clinically important, potentially hazardous interactions with: telithromycin

Reactions

Skin
 Allergic reactions (sic) [1]
 Edema (<1%)
 Exanthems (6%) [2]
 Fixed eruption (1%)
 Pruritus (>1%) [1]
 Rash (sic) (5%)
 Raynaud's phenomenon [1]
 Urticaria [2]

Hair
 Hair – pigmentation [2]

Cardiovascular
 Bradycardia [4]
 Flushing (>1%)

Other
 Anaphylactoid reactions (1–10%) [6]
 Cough [2]
 Death [4]
 Dysgeusia (<1%)
 Injection-site erythema (<1%)
 Injection-site pain (>10%) [26]
 Injection-site pruritus (<1%)
 Myalgia (>1%)
 Phlebitis
 Rhabdomyolysis [2]
 Seizures [1]
 Sialorrhea (>1%)
 Tinnitus
 Twitching (1–10%)
 Xerostomia (<1%)

PROTRIPTYLINE

Trade name: Vivactil (Odyssey)
Other common trade names: *Concordin; Triptil*
Indications: Depression
Category: Tricyclic antidepressant
Half-life: 54–92 hours
Clinically important, potentially hazardous interactions with: amprenavir, arbutamine, clonidine, epinephrine, formoterol, guanethidine, isocarboxazid, linezolid, MAO inhibitors, phenelzine, quinolones, sparfloxacin, tranylcypromine

Reactions

Skin
 Acne
 Allergic reactions (sic) (<1%)
 Angioedema
 Dermatitis (3%) [1]

 Diaphoresis (1–10%)
 Edema
 Erythema
 Exanthems
 Petechiae

Photosensitivity (<1%) [1]
Phototoxicity [1]
Pruritus (1–5%) [1]
Purpura
Rash (sic)
Urticaria
Vasculitis
Xerosis

Hair
Hair – alopecia (<1%)

Cardiovascular
Flushing

Other
Black tongue

Death
Dysgeusia (>10%)
Galactorrhea (<1%)
Glossitis
Gynecomastia (<1%)
Headache
Oral mucosal eruption
Paresthesias
Parkinsonism (1–10%)
Rhabdomyolysis [1]
Stomatitis
Tinnitus
Tremor
Xerostomia (>10%)

QUAZEPAM

Trade name: Doral (MedPointe)
Other common trade names: *Oniria; Pamerex; Quazium; Quiedorm; Selepam; Temodal*
Indications: Insomnia
Category: Antidepressant; Benzodiazepine sedative-hypnotic
Half-life: 25–41 hours
Clinically important, potentially hazardous interactions with: amprenavir,
chlorpheniramine, clarithromycin, efavirenz, esomeprazole, imatinib, indinavir, nelfinavir, ritonavir

---

Reactions

Skin
Dermatitis (1–10%)
Diaphoresis (>10%)
Pruritus [1]
Purpura
Rash (sic) (>10%) [1]
Urticaria

Hair
Hair – alopecia
Hair – hirsutism

Other
Dysgeusia
Headache
Oral ulceration
Paresthesias
Sialopenia (>10%)
Sialorrhea (1–10%)
Xerostomia (1–5%) [1]

QUETIAPINE

Trade name: Seroquel (AstraZeneca)
Indications: Psychotic disorders, schizophrenia
Category: Antipsychotic
Half-life: ~6 hours

Reactions

Skin
Angioedema [1]
Candidiasis (<1%)
Diaphoresis (1–10%)
Edema
Facial edema (<1%)
Neuroleptic malignant syndrome [5]
Photosensitivity (<1%)
Rash (sic) (4%)
Xerosis (<1%)

Cardiovascular
QT prolongation [1]

Other
Bruxism (<1%)

Gingivitis (<1%)
Glossitis (<1%)
Headache
Myalgia (<1%) [1]
Oral ulceration (<1%)
Paresthesias (1%)
Priapism [1]
Sialorrhea (<1%)
Stomatitis (<1%)
Thrombophlebitis (<1%)
Tic disorder [1]
Tongue edema (<1%)
Xerostomia (7–14%) [2]

RED CLOVER

Scientific name: *Trifolium pratense*
Family: Leguminosae
Trade and other common names: Coumestrol; Cow Clover; Cowgrass; Meadow Clover; Menoflavon (Pascoe); Pavine Clover; Promensil (Novogen); Purple Clover; Three-Leaved Grass
Category: Phytoestrogen
Purported indications and other uses: Menopausal symptoms, hot flashes, muscle spasms, hypercholesterolemia, breast pain, osteoporosis, diuretic, expectorant, mild antispasmodic, sedative, blood purifier, bladder infections, liver disorders. Ointment for acne, eczema, psoriasis and other rashes
Half-life: N/A
Clinically important, potentially hazardous interactions with: conjugated estrogens, heparin, ticlopidine, warfarin

Note: Red clover contains phytoestrogens that bind to estrogen and progesterone receptors, potentially adversely affecting breast tissue

Reactions

None

RESERPINE

Trade names: Resa; Ser-Ap-Es (Novartis); Serpalan; Serpasil (Novartis); Serpatabs
Other common trade names: *Anserpin; Inerpin; Novo-Reserpine; Reserfia; Sedaraupin; Serpasol; Tionsera*
Indications: Hypertension
Category: Nondiuretic antihypertensive; Rauwolfia alkaloid
Half-life: 50–100 hours
Clinically important, potentially hazardous interactions with: metipranolol

Ser-Ap-Es is reserpine, hydralazine and hydrochlorothiazide

Reactions

Skin
  Bullous eruption [1]
  Edema
  Exanthems
  Lupus erythematosus (exacerbation) [1]
  Peripheral edema (1–10%)
  Pruritus
  Purpura
  Rash (sic) (<1%)
  Toxic epidermal necrolysis [1]
  Urticaria

Cardiovascular
  Bradycardia [1]
  Flushing

Other
  Gynecomastia
  Headache
  Parkinsonism
  Sialorrhea
  Xerostomia (>10%)

RISPERIDONE

Trade name: Risperdal (Janssen)
Indications: Psychotic disorders
Category: Antipsychotic
Half-life: 3–30 hours
Clinically important, potentially hazardous interactions with: clozapine, paroxetine

Reactions

Skin
  Acne (<1%)
  Allergic reactions (sic) (<1%) [1]
  Angioedema [2]
  Bullous eruption (<1%)
  Bullous pemphigoid [1]
  Dermatitis
  Diaphoresis (<1%)
  Edema [2]
  Exfoliative dermatitis (0.1–1%)
  Furunculosis (<1%)
  Hyperkeratosis (<1%)
  Hypohidrosis (<1%)
  Irritation (sic) (22%) [1]
  Lichenoid eruption (<1%)
  Neuroleptic malignant syndrome [5]
  Peripheral edema (16%) [1]
  Photosensitivity (1–10%) [1]
  Pigmentation (1%)
  Pruritus (<1%)

Psoriasis (<1%)
Purpura (<1%)
Rash (sic) (5%)
Seborrhea
Ulcerations (<1%)
Urticaria (<0.1%)
Warts (<1%)
Xerosis (2%)

Hair
Hair – alopecia (<1%) [1]
Hair – hypertrichosis (<1%)

Cardiovascular
Flushing (<1%) [1]
QT prolongation [1]

Other
Akathisia [1]
Anaphylactoid reactions
Anxiety (24%) [1]
Death
Depression (14%) [3]
Dysgeusia (<1%)
Dysphagia [2]
Galactorrhea (1–10%) [2]
Gingivitis (<1%)

Gynecomastia (1–10%) [1]
Headache
Hyperesthesia (<1%)
Mastodynia (<1%)
Muscle rigidity (10%) [1]
Myalgia (<1%)
Paresthesias (<1%)
Parkinsonism [1]
Priapism (1–10%) [5]
Psychosis [1]
Restless legs syndrome [1]
Rhabdomyolysis [2]
Seizures [1]
Sialopenia (5%)
Sialorrhea (2%) [1]
Stomatitis (<1%)
Stutter [1]
Tardive dyskinesia [1]
Thrombophlebitis (<1%)
Tinnitus
Tongue edema (<1%)
Tongue pigmentation (<1%)
Tremor (14%) [1]
Xerostomia (1–18%) [3]

RIVASTIGMINE

Trade name: Exelon (Novartis)
Indications: Alzheimer's disease and dementia
Category: Acetylcholinesterase inhibitor; Cholinergic
Half-life: 1–2 hours
Clinically important, potentially hazardous interactions with: galantamine

Reactions

Skin
Allergic reactions (sic) (~1%)
Bullous eruption (~1%)
Cellulitis (~1%)
Clammy skin (~1%)
Dermatitis (~1%)
Diaphoresis (10%)
Edema (~1%)

Exanthems (~1%) [1]
Exfoliative dermatitis (~1%)
Facial edema (~1%)
Herpes simplex (~1%)
Infections (~2%)
Peripheral edema (~2%)
Psoriasis (~1%)
Purpura (~1%)

Rash (sic) (~2%)
Ulcerations (~1%)
Urticaria (~1%)

Hair
Hair – alopecia (~1%)

Eyes
Periorbital edema (~1%)

Cardiovascular
Flushing (~1%)
Hot flashes (~1%)

Other
Ageusia (~1%)
Dysgeusia (~1%)

Foetor ex ore (halitosis) (~1%)
Gingivitis (~1%)
Glossitis (~1%)
Headache
Hyperesthesia (~1%)
Mastodynia (~1%)
Myalgia (20%)
Paresthesias (~1%)
Sialorrhea (~1%)
Thrombophlebitis (<2%)
Tremor (4%)
Ulcerative stomatitis (~1%)
Vaginitis (~1%)
Xerostomia (~1%)

SECOBARBITAL

Synonym: quinalbarbitone
Trade name: Seconal (Ranbaxy)
Other common trade names: *Immenoctal; Novo-Secobarb; Secanal*
Indications: Insomnia
Category: Short-acting barbiturate sedative-hypnotic
Half-life: 15–40 hours
Clinically important, potentially hazardous interactions with: alcohol, anticoagulants, antihistamines, brompheniramine, buclizine, chlorpheniramine, dicumarol, ethanolamine, imatinib, warfarin

Reactions

Skin
Angioedema (<1%)
Exanthems
Exfoliative dermatitis (<1%)
Purpura
Rash (sic) (<1%)
Stevens–Johnson syndrome (<1%)
Urticaria

Other
Headache
Hypersensitivity
Injection-site pain (>10%)
Rhabdomyolysis [1]
Serum sickness
Thrombophlebitis (<1%)

SELEGILINE

Synonyms: deprenyl; L-deprenyl
Trade name: Eldepryl (Somerset)
Other common trade names: *Apo-Selegiline; Carbex; Eldeprine; Jumex; Movergan; Novo-Selegiline; Plurimen*
Indications: Parkinsonism
Category: Antiparkinsonian; Monoamine oxidase (MAO) inhibitor
Half-life: 9 minutes
Clinically important, potentially hazardous interactions with: carbidopa, carbidopa, citalopram, doxepin, **ephedra**, ephedrine, escitalopram, fluoxetine, fluvoxamine, levodopa, meperidine, nefazodone, oral contraceptives, paroxetine, sertraline, venlafaxine

Reactions

Skin
  Diaphoresis
  Peripheral edema
  Photosensitivity
  Rash (sic)

Hair
  Hair – alopecia
  Hair – hypertrichosis (facial)

Other
  Application-site reactions (sic) [1]
  Bruxism (1–10%)

Death [1]
Dysgeusia
Headache
Oral ulceration [1]
Paresthesias
Serotonin syndrome [1]
Stomatitis [1]
Tinnitus
Tremor
Xerostomia (>10%) [1]

SERTRALINE

Trade name: Zoloft (Pfizer)
Other common trade name: *Atruline*
Indications: Depression, panic disorders, obsessive compulsive disorders
Category: Antidepressant; Selective serotonin reuptake inhibitor (SSRI)
Half-life: 24–26 hours
Clinically important, potentially hazardous interactions with: amphetamines, clarithromycin, dextroamphetamine, diethylpropion, erythromycin, isocarboxazid, linezolid, MAO inhibitors*, mazindol, methamphetamine, metoclopramide, phendimetrazine, phenelzine, phentermine, phenylpropanolamine, pimozide, pseudoephedrine, selegiline, sibutramine, **St John's wort**, sumatriptan, sympathomimetics, tranylcypromine, trazodone, troleandomycin

Reactions

Skin
  Acne (<1%)

Allergic reactions (sic) [2]
Angioedema [2]

Balanitis (<1%)
Bullous eruption (<1%) [1]
Dermatitis (<1%)
Diaphoresis (8.4%) [6]
Discoloration (<1%)
Edema (<1%)
Erythema
Erythema multiforme (<1%) [1]
Exanthems (<1%) [4]
Fixed eruption [1]
Lupus erythematosus [1]
Necrosis [1]
Night sweats [1]
Photosensitivity (<1%)
Pruritus (<1%) [1]
Purpura (<1%)
Rash (sic) (2.1%)
Stevens–Johnson syndrome [1]
Urticaria (<1%)
Xerosis (<1%)

Hair

Hair – abnormal texture (<1%)
Hair – alopecia (<1%) [1]
Hair – hirsutism (<1%)

Eyes

Periorbital edema (<1%)

Cardiovascular

Flushing (2.2%)

QT prolongation [1]

Other

Akathisia [1]
Aphthous stomatitis (<1%)
Bromhidrosis (<1%)
Bruxism (<1%)
Death [4]
Dysgeusia
Dystonia [1]
Foetor ex ore (halitosis) (<1%)
Galactorrhea [1]
Gingival hypertrophy (<1%)
Glossitis (<1%)
Gynecomastia (<1%)
Headache
Hyperesthesia (<1%)
Paresthesias (2%)
Priapism [1]
Serotonin syndrome [5]
Sialorrhea (<1%)
Stomatitis (<1%)
Tinnitus
Tongue edema (<1%)
Tongue ulceration (<1%)
Tremor (1–10%) [1]
Vaginitis (atrophic)
Xerostomia (16.3%) [5]

SIBERIAN GINSENG

Scientific names: *Acanthopanax senticosus; Eleutherococcus senticosus*
Family: Araliaceae
Trade and other common names: Ciwuija; Devil's root; Eleuthero; Ezoukogi; Medexport; Shigoka; Taiga Wurzel; Touch-me-not
Category: Adaptogen; Antidementia; Emmenagogue; Immunoregulator
Purported indications and other uses: Alzheimer's disease, anaphylaxis, arthritis, colds, depression, fatigue, flu, impotence, infertility, menopause, multiple sclerosis, osteoporosis, perimenopause, PMS, stress
Half-life: N/A
Clinically important, potentially hazardous interactions with: antihypertensives, digoxin

Reactions

Other   Mastodynia
  Headache
Note: Eleutherococcus may prevent biotransformation of some drugs to less toxic compounds

SIBUTRAMINE

Trade name: Meridia (Abbott)
Indications: Obesity
Category: Anorexiant; Obesity management
Half-life: 1.1 hours
Clinically important, potentially hazardous interactions with: dextromethorphan, dihydroergotamine, **ephedra**, ergot, fluoxetine, fluvoxamine, isocarboxazid, linezolid, lithium, MAO inhibitors, meperidine, methysergide, naratriptan, nefazodone, paroxetine, phenelzine, rizatriptan, sertraline, sumatriptan, tranylcypromine, **tryptophan**, venlafaxine, verapamil, zolmitriptan

Reactions

Skin
  Acne (1.0%)
  Allergic reactions (sic) (1.5%)
  Diaphoresis (2.5%)
  Edema (2%)
  Flu-like syndrome (1–10%)
  Herpes simplex (1.3%)
  Peripheral edema (>1%)
  Pruritus (>1%)
  Rash (sic) (3.8%)
  Xerosis [1]

Hematopoietic
  Ecchymoses (0.7%)

Cardiovascular
  QT prolongation [1]

Other
  Death [1]
  Dysgeusia (2.2%)
  Headache [1]
  Myalgia (1.9%)
  Paresthesias (2.0%)
  Tooth disorder (sic)
  Vulvovaginal candidiasis (1.2%)
  Xerostomia (17.2%) [2]

SODIUM OXYBATE

Synonyms: Gamma Hydroxybutyrate; GHB
Trade name: Xyrem (Orphan Medical)
Indications: Cataplexy (in patients with narcolepsy)
Category: Anesthetic; Anticataplectic; CNS depressant; Dietary supplement
Half-life: 0.3–1 hour
Clinically important, potentially hazardous interactions with: alcohol, hypnotics, sedatives

Reactions

Skin
Diaphoresis [3]
Flu-like syndrome
Infections
Upper respiratory infection

Other
Back pain
Death [9]

Depression
Pain
Porphyria
Rhabdomyolysis
Seizures [7]
Sialorrhea
Sinusitis
Tremor [4]

Note: Sodium Oxybate is a class of drugs that are also known as: 'Designer' drugs; Party drugs; Club drugs; Recreational drugs; 'Rave' drugs; Fantasy drugs; Date rape drugs; abuse drugs

ST JOHN'S WORT

Scientific name: *Hypericum perforatum*
Family: Hypericaceae
Trade and other common names: Amber; Demon Chaser; Fuga Daemonum; Goatweed; Hardhay; Hypereikon; Hypericum; Johns Wort; Klamath Weed; Rosin Rose; Tipton Weed
Category: Anti-anxiety
Purported indications and other uses: Depression, dysthymic disorder, fatigue, insomnia, loss of appetite, anxiety, obsessive-compulsive disorders, mood disturbances, migraine headaches, neuralgia, fibrositis, sciatica, palpitations, exhaustion, headache, muscle pain, vitiligo, diuretic, bruises, abrasions, first degree burns, hemorrhoids
Half-life: N/A
Clinically important, potentially hazardous interactions with: alprazolam, amitriptyline, amprenavir, atazanavir, bosentan, buspirone, carbamazepine, citalopram, cyclosporine, digoxin, eplerenone, escitalopram, etoposide, fexofenadine, fluoxetine, fluvoxamine, fosamprenavir, **ginkgo biloba**, imatinib, indinavir, irinotecan, loperamide, methadone, midazolam, naratriptan, nefazodone, nelfinavir, nevirapine, oral contraceptives, paroxetine, phenobarbitone, phenprocoumon, phenytoin, quinolones ritonavir, ritonavir, rizatriptan, saquinavir, sertraline, simvastatin, sirolimus, solifenacin, SSRIs, sumatriptan, tacrolimus, tetracyclines, theophylline, tricyclic antidepressants, warfarin, zolmitriptan

Reactions

Skin
Adverse effects (sic) [2]
Allergic reactions (sic) [1]
Erythroderma [1]
Irritation
Photosensitivity [6]
Pruritus [1]

Hair
Hair – alopecia [1]

Other
Bleeding [1]
Hypersensitivity
Paresthesias [1]
Serotonin syndrome [4]
Side effects (sic) [1]
Xerostomia [1]

Note: St. John's wort is a natural source of flavoring in Europe. Although not indigenous to Australia, and long considered a weed, St. John's wort is now grown there as a cash crop and produces 20% of the world's supply

SUMATRIPTAN

Trade name: Imitrex (GSK)
Other common trade name: *Imigrane*
Indications: Migraine attacks
Category: Antimigraine; Serotonin agonist
Half-life: 2.5 hours
Clinically important, potentially hazardous interactions with: citalopram, dihydroergotamine, ergot-containing drugs, escitalopram, fluoxetine, fluvoxamine, isocarboxazid, MAO inhibitors*, methysergide, naratriptan, nefazodone, paroxetine, phenelzine, rizatriptan, sertraline, sibutramine, **St John's wort**, tranylcypromine, venlafaxine, zolmitriptan

Reactions

Skin
Angioedema [1]
Burning (1–10%)
Diaphoresis (1.6%)
Erythema (<1%)
Exanthems
Hyperpyrexia [1]
Photosensitivity (<1%)
Pruritus (<1%)
Rash (sic) (<1%)
Raynaud's phenomenon (<1%)
Sensitivity (sic) [1]
Urticaria [1]

Cardiovascular
Atrial fibrillation [1]
Coronary artery disorders [1]
Flushing (6.6%)
Hot flashes (>10%)
Myocardial ischemia [1]

Other
Anaphylactoid reactions
Dysesthesia (<1%)
Dysgeusia (<1%) [1]
Glossodynia
Headache
Hyperesthesia (<1%)
Injection-site reactions (sic) (10–58%) [1]

Myalgia (1.8%)
Parageusia (<1%)
Paresthesias (13.5%)

Parosmia (<1%)
Xerostomia

TACRINE

Synonym: THA
Trade name: Cognex (First Horizon)
Indications: Dementia of Alzheimer's disease
Category: Anticholinesterase; Cholinergic
Half-life: 1.5–4 hours
Clinically important, potentially hazardous interactions with: fluvoxamine, galantamine

Reactions

Skin
 Acne (<1%)
 Basal cell carcinoma
 Bullous eruption
 Cellulitis
 Cyst
 Dermatitis (<1%)
 Desquamation
 Diaphoresis
 Eczema
 Edema (<1%)
 Exanthems (7%)
 Facial edema (<1%)
 Furunculosis (<1%)
 Herpes simplex (<1%)
 Herpes zoster (<1%)
 Melanoma (<1%)
 Necrosis (<1%)
 Peripheral edema (<1%)
 Petechiae
 Pruritus (7%)
 Psoriasis (<1%)
 Purpura (2%)
 Rash (sic) (7%)

 Seborrhea
 Squamous cell carcinoma
 Ulcerations (<1%)
 Urticaria (7%)
 Xerosis (<1%)

Hair
 Hair – alopecia (<1%)

Cardiovascular
 Bradycardia [1]
 Flushing (3%)

Other
 Dysgeusia (<1%)
 Gingivitis (<1%)
 Glossitis (<1%)
 Headache
 Myalgia (9%)
 Paresthesias (<1%)
 Parkinsonism [1]
 Sialorrhea (<1%)
 Stomatitis (<1%)
 Tremor (1–10%)
 Xerostomia (<1%)

TEMAZEPAM

Trade names: Restoril (Mallinckrodt); Temazepam
Other common trade names: *Apo-Temazepam; Cerepax; Euhypnos; Lenal; Levanxene; Normison; Nu-Temazepam; Planum*
Indications: Insomnia, anxiety
Category: Benzodiazepine sedative-hypnotic
Half-life: 8–15 hours
Clinically important, potentially hazardous interactions with: amprenavir, chlorpheniramine, clarithromycin, efavirenz, esomeprazole, imatinib, nelfinavir

Reactions

Skin
Adverse effects (sic) [1]
Bullous eruption [1]
Dermatitis (1–10%)
Diaphoresis (>10%)
Exanthems
Fixed eruption [1]
Lichenoid eruption [1]
Pruritus
Purpura
Rash (sic) (>10%)
Urticaria

Other
Anaphylactoid reactions [1]
Dysgeusia
Headache
Paresthesias
Sialopenia (>10%)
Sialorrhea (1–10%)
Tremor (<1%)
Xerostomia (1.7%)

THIOPENTAL

Trade name: Thiopental (Baxter)
Other common trade names: *Anesthal; Hypnostan; Intraval; Nesdonal; Sodipental; Trapanal*
Indications: Induction of anesthesia
Category: Anticonvulsant; Barbiturate anesthetic; Sedative
Half-life: 3–12 hours
Clinically important, potentially hazardous interactions with: ethanol, ethanolamine

Reactions

Skin
Angioedema [4]
Bullous eruption [2]
Erythema (<1%)
Erythema multiforme [2]
Exanthems (3%) [3]
Exfoliative dermatitis
Fixed eruption [3]
Hypomelanosis [1]
Pruritus (<1%)
Purpura [2]
Rash (sic)
Shivering (27%) [1]
Stevens–Johnson syndrome [1]
Toxic epidermal necrolysis [1]
Urticaria [4]

Other
Anaphylactoid reactions (<1%) [9]

Headache
Injection-site necrosis
Injection-site pain (>10%)
Injection-site phlebitis (6%) [1]

Porphyria [4]
Rhabdomyolysis [1]
Thrombophlebitis (<1%)
Twitching (<1%)

THIORIDAZINE

Trade name: Mellaril (Novartis)
Other common trade names: *Aldazine; Apo-Thioridazine; Calmaril; Dazine; Melleril; Ridazin; Thinin; Thioril*
Indications: Psychotic disorders
Category: Phenothiazine antipsychotic
Half-life: 21–25 hours
Clinically important, potentially hazardous interactions with: antihistamines, arsenic, chlorpheniramine, dofetilide, duloxetine, epinephrine, **evening primrose**, pimozide, piperazine, quinolones, sparfloxacin, telithromycin

Reactions

Skin
Acanthosis nigricans [1]
Angioedema (<1%) [1]
Dermatitis [1]
Erythema multiforme [1]
Exanthems [1]
Exfoliative dermatitis
Hypohidrosis (>10%)
Lupus erythematosus [1]
Peripheral edema
Photosensitivity (1–10%) [2]
Phototoxicity [2]
Pigmentation (<1%) (blue-gray) [2]
Purpura
Rash (sic) (1–10%) [3]
Seborrhea
Toxic epidermal necrolysis [1]
Urticaria
Vasculitis [1]
Xerosis

Hair
Hair – alopecia
Hair – hypertrichosis [1]

Eyes
Retinopathy [1]

Cardiovascular
Arrhythmias [1]
QT prolongation [2]
Tachycardia [1]

Other
Anaphylactoid reactions
Death [2]
Galactorrhea (<1%)
Gynecomastia
Headache
Hypersensitivity
Lymphoproliferative disease [1]
Mastodynia (1–10%)
Oral mucosal eruption [1]
Paresthesias
Parkinsonism (>10%)
Parotitis [1]
Porphyria [1]
Priapism (<1%) [1]
Pseudolymphoma [1]
Tardive dyskinesia [1]
Tremor
Xerostomia [1]

THIOTHIXENE

Synonym: tiotixene
Trade name: Navane (Pfizer)
Other common trade name: *Orbinamon*
Indications: Psychotic disorders
Category: Antipsychotic
Half-life: >24 hours

Reactions

Skin
Diaphoresis (14%) [1]
Exanthems (14%) [2]
Hypohidrosis (>10%)
Palmar erythema [1]
Peripheral edema
Photosensitivity (1–10%) [2]
Pigmentation (blue-gray) (<1%)
Pruritus
Rash (sic) (1–10%)
Raynaud's phenomenon [1]
Seborrheic dermatitis [2]
Sensitivity (sic) [1]
Telangiectasia [1]
Urticaria

Hair
Hair – alopecia

Other
Anaphylactoid reactions
Black tongue [1]
Dysgeusia [1]
Galactorrhea (<1%)
Gynecomastia
Mastodynia (1–10%)
Paresthesias
Parkinsonism (>10%)
Priapism (<1%)
Sialorrhea
Xerostomia [2]

TIAGABINE

Trade name: Gabitril (Cephalon)
Indications: Partial seizures
Category: Anticonvulsant
Half-life: 7–9 hours

Reactions

Skin
Acne (>1%)
Allergic reactions (sic) (<1%)
Carcinoma (<1%)
Dermatitis (<1%)
Diaphoresis (<1%)
Eczema (<1%)
Edema (<1%)
Exanthems (<1%)
Exfoliative dermatitis (<1%)
Facial edema (<1%)
Furunculosis (<1%)
Herpes simplex (<1%)
Herpes zoster (<1%)
Neoplasms (benign) (<1%)
Nodular eruption (<1%)

Peripheral edema (<1%)
Petechiae (<1%)
Photosensitivity (<1%)
Pigmentation (<1%)
Pruritus (2%)
Psoriasis (<1%)
Rash (sic) (5%)
Stevens–Johnson syndrome
Ulcerations (<1%)
Urticaria (<1%)
Vesiculobullous eruption (<1%)
Xerosis (<1%)

Hair
Hair – alopecia (<1%)
Hair – hirsutism (<1%)

Hematopoietic
Ecchymoses (>1%)

Other
Ageusia (<1%)

Depression [1]
Dysgeusia (<1%)
Foetor ex ore (halitosis) (<1%)
Gingival hypertrophy (<1%)
Gingivitis (<1%)
Glossitis (<1%)
Gynecomastia (<1%)
Mastodynia (<1%)
Myalgia (>1%)
Oral ulceration (2%)
Paresthesias (4%)
Parosmia (<1%)
Sialorrhea (<1%)
Stomatitis (<1%)
Thrombophlebitis (<1%)
Tremor (>1%) [2]
Ulcerative stomatitis (<1%)
Vaginitis (<1%)
Xerostomia (>1%)

TOPIRAMATE

Trade name: Topamax (Ortho-McNeil)
Indications: Partial onset seizures
Category: Anticonvulsant
Half-life: 21 hours

Reactions

Skin
Acne (>1%)
Basal cell carcinoma (<1%)
Dermatitis (<1%)
Diaphoresis (1.8%)
Eczema (<1%)
Edema (1.8%)
Exanthems (<1%) [1]
Facial edema (<1%) [1]
Flu-like syndrome (1–10%)
Folliculitis (<1%)
Hypohidrosis (<1%) [2]
Palmar erythema [1]
Photosensitivity (<1%)
Pigmentation (<1%)

Pruritus (1.8%) [1]
Purpura (<1%)
Rash (sic) (4.4%)
Seborrhea (<1%)
Urticaria (<1%)
Xerosis (<1%)

Hair
Hair – abnormal texture (<1%)
Hair – alopecia (>1%) [1]

Nails
Nails – changes (sic) (<1%)

Eyes
Blurred vision [1]

Glaucoma [4]
Myopia [3]
Periorbital edema [1]
Scleritis [1]

Cardiovascular
Flushing (<1%)
Hot flashes (1–10%)

Other
Ageusia (<1%)
Bromhidrosis (1.8%)
Depression [3]
Dizziness (6%) [2]
Dysgeusia (>1%) [3]
Fatigue [2]
Foetor ex ore (halitosis)

Gingival hypertrophy (<1%)
Gingivitis (1.8%)
Gynecomastia (8.3%)
Hyperesthesia (<1%)
Mastodynia (3–9%)
Myalgia (1.8%)
Oligohydrosis [1]
Paresthesias (15%) [11]
Parosmia (<1%)
Seizures [1]
Sialorrhea [1]
Stomatitis (<1%)
Tongue edema (<1%)
Tremor (>10%)
Vaginitis
Xerostomia (2.7%)

TRANYLCYPROMINE

Trade name: Parnate
Other common trade name: *Siciton*
Indications: Depression
Category: Antidepressant; Monoamine oxidase (MAO) inhibitor
Half-life: 2.5 hours
Clinically important, potentially hazardous interactions with: amitriptyline, amoxapine, amphetamines, bupropion, citalopram, clomipramine, cyproheptadine, desipramine, dextroamphetamine, dextromethorphan, diethylpropion, dopamine, doxepin, entacapone, ephedrine, epinephrine, fluoxetine, fluvoxamine, imipramine, levodopa, mazindol, meperidine, methamphetamine, nefazodone, nortriptyline, paroxetine, phendimetrazine, phentermine, phenylephrine, phenylpropanolamine, protriptyline, pseudoephedrine, rizatriptan, sertraline, sibutramine, sumatriptan, sympathomimetics, tramadol, tricyclic antidepressants, trimipramine, **tryptophan, tyramine-containing foods***, venlafaxine, zolmitriptan

Reactions

Skin
Diaphoresis [1]
Edema (<1%)
Exanthems
Neuroleptic malignant syndrome [1]
Peripheral edema
Photosensitivity (<1%)
Pruritus
Rash (sic) (<1%)

Urticaria

Cardiovascular
Atrial fibrillation [1]
Flushing [1]

Other
Acute intermittent porphyria [1]
Black tongue
Headache
Paresthesias

Priapism
Rhabdomyolysis [1]
Tinnitus

Tremor
Twitching
Xerostomia (<1%)

*Note: Tyramine-containing foods include the following: aged cheeses, avocados, banana skins, bologna and other processed luncheon meats, chicken livers, chocolate, figs, canned pickled herring, meat extracts, pepperoni, raisins, raspberries, soy sauce, vermouth, sherry and red wines

TRAZODONE

Trade name: Desyrel (Bristol-Myers Squibb)
Other common trade names: *Alti-Trazodone; Bimaran; Deprax; Desirel; Molipaxin; Sideril; Taxagon; Trazalon*
Indications: Depression
Category: Heterocyclic antidepressant
Half-life: 3–6 hours
Clinically important, potentially hazardous interactions with: citalopram, fluoxetine, fluvoxamine, **ginkgo biloba**, linezolid, nefazodone, paroxetine, sertraline, venlafaxine

Reactions

Skin
Angioedema [1]
Diaphoresis (>1%)
Edema (1–10%)
Erythema multiforme [1]
Exanthems [6]
Exfoliative dermatitis [1]
Formication [1]
Photosensitivity [2]
Pruritus (<1%)
Psoriasis (exacerbation) [2]
Purpura
Rash (sic) (<1%) [1]
Urticaria [3]
Vasculitis [1]

Hair
Hair – alopecia [2]

Nails
Nails – leukonychia [1]

Cardiovascular
Atrial fibrillation [1]
Bradycardia [1]

Other
Dysgeusia (>10%)
Dysphagia [1]
Galactorrhea
Gynecomastia
Headache
Hypersensitivity
Myalgia (1–10%)
Paresthesias (>1%)
Parkinsonism [1]
Priapism (12%) [7]
Serotonin syndrome [3]
Sialorrhea
Tremor (1–10%)
Xerostomia (>10%) [1]

TRIAZOLAM

Trade name: Halcion (Pfizer)
Other common trade names: *Dumozolam; Novo-Triolam; Nu-Triazo; Nuctane; Somese; Somniton; Songar; Trialam*
Indications: Insomnia
Category: Benzodiazepine sedative-hypnotic
Half-life: 1.5–5.5 hours
Clinically important, potentially hazardous interactions with: atazanavir, clarithromycin, delavirdine, efavirenz, erythromycin, fosamprenavir, indinavir, itraconazole, ketoconazole, rifampin, ritonavir, telithromycin

Reactions

Skin
Dermatitis (1–10%) [1]
Diaphoresis (>10%) [2]
Exanthems
Photosensitivity [1]
Pruritus [2]
Purpura
Rash (sic) (>10%) [1]
Urticaria

Hair
Hair – alopecia
Hair – hirsutism

Other
Dysesthesia (<1%)

Dysgeusia (<1%) [2]
Gingivitis
Glossitis (<1%)
Glossodynia (<1%)
Headache
Paresthesias (<1%) [1]
Sialopenia (>10%) [1]
Sialorrhea (1–10%)
Stomatitis (<1%)
Tinnitus
Tremor (1–10%)
Xerostomia (>10%) [4]

TRIFLUOPERAZINE

Trade name: Stelazine
Other common trade names: *Calmazine; Domilium; Flupazine; Fluzine; Nerolet; Psyrazine; Sedizine; Tfp*
Indications: Psychoses, anxiety
Category: Antipsychotic; Anxiolytic; Phenothiazine tranquilizer
Half-life: 10–20 hours
Clinically important, potentially hazardous interactions with: antihistamines, arsenic, chlorpheniramine, dofetilide, piperazine, quinolones, sparfloxacin

Reactions

Skin
Angioedema [1]

Dermatitis
Diaphoresis

Eczema
Erythema
Exanthems
Exfoliative dermatitis
Fixed eruption [1]
Hypohidrosis
Lupus erythematosus
Neuroleptic malignant syndrome [1]
Peripheral edema
Photosensitivity (1–10%) [1]
Pigmentation (blue-gray) (<1%) [1]
Pruritus
Purpura
Rash (sic) (1–10%)
Seborrhea
Urticaria

Xerosis

Other
Anaphylactoid reactions
Galactorrhea (<1%)
Gynecomastia
Headache
Mastodynia (1–10%)
Oral mucosal eruption [1]
Parkinsonism (>10%)
Priapism (<1%)
Rhabdomyolysis [1]
Tongue edema [1]
Tremor
Xerostomia

TRIMEPRAZINE

Trade name: Temaril
Other common trade names: *Nedeltran; Panectyl; Theralene; Vallergan; Variargil*
Indications: Pruritus, urticaria
Category: Antihistamine; Phenothiazine tranquilizer
Duration of action: 3–6 hours

Reactions

Skin
Angioedema (<1%) [1]
Dermatitis
Diaphoresis
Edema (<1%)
Exanthems [1]
Lupus erythematosus
Peripheral edema
Photosensitivity (<1%)
Pruritus [1]
Purpura

Rash (sic) (<1%)
Urticaria

Other
Anaphylactoid reactions
Gynecomastia
Myalgia (<1%)
Paresthesias (<1%)
Stomatitis
Tinnitus
Xerostomia (1–10%) [1]

TRIMETHADIONE

Trade name: Tridione
Other common trade name: *Mino Aleviatin*
Category: Anticonvulsant
Half-life: N/A

Reactions

Skin
 Acne
 Bullous eruption
 Erythema multiforme [4]
 Exanthems [3]
 Exfoliative dermatitis [2]
 Fixed eruption
 Infections (3%) [1]
 Lupus erythematosus [6]
 Petechiae
 Photosensitivity [1]
 Pruritus [1]
 Purpura [1]

 Stevens–Johnson syndrome [1]
 Urticaria [3]
 Vasculitis [2]

Hair
 Hair – alopecia [1]

Other
 Acute intermittent porphyria
 Gingivitis
 Mucositis (4%) [1]
 Paresthesias

TRIMETHOBENZAMIDE

Trade names: Arrestin; Benzacot; Bio-Gan; Navogan; Stemetic; T-Gene; Tebamide; Tegamide; Ticon; Tigan (Monarch); Triban; Tribenzagen; Trimazide
Other common trade names: *Anaus; Elen; Ibikin*
Indications: Prevention and treatment of nausea and vomiting
Category: Antiemetic
Half-life: N/A

Reactions

Skin
 Allergic reactions (sic) (<1%)

Other
 Headache

 Hypersensitivity (<1%)
 Injection-site reactions (sic)
 Parkinsonism

TRIMIPRAMINE

Trade name: Surmontil (Odyssey)
Other common trade names: *Apo-Trimip; Rhotrimine; Stangyl; Sumontil*
Indications: Major depression
Category: Antineuralgic; Tricyclic antidepressant
Half-life: 20–26 hours
Clinically important, potentially hazardous interactions with: amprenavir, arbutamine, bupropion, clonidine, epinephrine, formoterol, guanethidine, isocarboxazid, linezolid, MAO inhibitors, phenelzine, quinolones, sparfloxacin, tranylcypromine

Reactions

Skin

Allergic reactions (sic) (<1%)
Diaphoresis (1–10%)
Exanthems
Petechiae
Photosensitivity (<1%)
Pruritus
Purpura
Rash (sic)
Urticaria

Hair

Hair – alopecia (<1%)

Cardiovascular

QT prolongation [1]

Other

Dysgeusia (>10%)
Galactorrhea (<1%)
Glossitis
Gynecomastia (<1%)
Paresthesias
Parkinsonism (1–10%)
Seizures [1]
Stomatitis
Tinnitus
Tremor
Xerostomia (>10%)

TRYPTOPHAN

Scientific name: *L-2-amino-3-(indole-3yl) propionic acid*
Family: None
Trade and other common names: 5-HT; 5-HTP; 5-hydroxytryptophan; 5-OHTrp; L-trypt; L-tryptophan
Category: Sedative; Serotonin modulator
Purported indications and other uses: Insomnia, depression, myofascial pain, premenstrual syndrome, smoking cessation, bruxism
Half-life: N/A
Clinically important, potentially hazardous interactions with: fluoxetine, fluvoxamine, isocarboxazid, phenelzine, sibutramine, tranylcypromine

Reactions

Skin
  Diaphoresis (with phenelzine)
  Scleroderma [4]

Other
  Death [1]

Eosinophilia–myalgia syndrome [17]
Fever [1]
Parkinsonism
Serotonin syndrome [1]
Shivering (with phenelzine)

Note: Tryptophan is an essential amino acid. It is a precursor of serotonin and is also converted to nicotinic acid and nicotinamide

VALERIAN

Scientific names: *Valeriana edulis; Valeriana jatamansii; Valeriana officinalis; Valeriana sitchensis; Valeriana wallichii*
Family: Valerianaceae
Trade and other common names: All-Heal; Amantilla; Baldrian; Garden Heliotrope
Category: Anxiolytic; Sedative-hypnotic
Purported indications and other uses: Depression, tremors, epilepsy, attention deficit hyperactivity disorder, rheumatism, nervous asthma, gastric spasms, colic, menstrual cramps, hot flashes. Flavoring in foods and beverages
Half-life: N/A
Clinically important, potentially hazardous interactions with: escitalopram

Reactions

Skin
  Adverse effects (sic) [1]

Other
  Toxicity [1]
  Tremor [1]

VALPROIC ACID

Trade names: Depacon (Abbott); Depakene (Abbott)
Indications: Seizures, migraine
Category: Anticonvulsant
Half-life: 6–16 hours
Clinically important, potentially hazardous interactions with: aspirin, cholestyramine, ivermectin

Reactions

Skin
  Acne
  Allergic reactions (sic) (<5%)
  Anticonvulsant hypersensitivity syndrome [3]
  Bullous eruption [1]
  Dermatitis
  Diaphoresis [1]
  Edema [1]
  Erythema multiforme (<1%) [2]
  Exanthems (5%) [1]
  Facial edema (>5%)
  Fixed eruption [1]
  Furunculosis (<5%)
  Lupus erythematosus [5]
  Morphea [1]
  Peripheral edema (<5%)
  Petechiae (<5%) [1]
  Photosensitivity [1]
  Pruritus (>5%) [1]
  Psoriasis
  Purpura [2]
  Rash (sic) (>5%) [2]
  Scleroderma [1]
  Seborrhea
  Stevens–Johnson syndrome [2]
  Toxic epidermal necrolysis [2]
  Urticaria
  Vasculitis [2]

Hair
  Hair – alopecia (7%) [13]
  Hair – curly [3]
  Hair – depigmentation [1]

Hematopoietic
  Ecchymoses (<5%) [4]

Other
  Acute intermittent porphyria [2]
  Aplasia cutis congenita
  Death [2]
  Dysgeusia (<5%)
  Galactorrhea [1]
  Gingival hypertrophy [3]
  Glossitis (<5%)
  Gynecomastia [1]
  Headache
  Hyperesthesia
  Hypersensitivity [3]
  Myalgia (<5%)
  Paresthesias (<5%)
  Parkinsonism [2]
  Porphyria [2]
  Pseudolymphoma [1]
  Rhabdomyolysis [1]
  Seizures [1]
  Sialorrhea
  Stomatitis (<5%)
  Tinnitus [1]
  Tremor [3]
  Vaginitis (<5%)
  Xerostomia (<5%) [1]

VENLAFAXINE

Trade name: Effexor (Wyeth)
Indications: Depression
Category: Heterocyclic antidepressant; Selective serotonin reuptake inhibitor (SSRI)
Half-life: 3–7 hours
Clinically important, potentially hazardous interactions with: isocarboxazid, linezolid, MAO inhibitors, metoclopramide, phenelzine, selegiline, sibutramine, sumatriptan, telithromycin, tramadol, tranylcypromine, trazodone

Reactions

Skin
Acne (<1%)
Allergic reactions (sic) (<1%)
Candidiasis
Dermatitis
Diaphoresis [1]
Eczema (<1%)
Edema (<1%)
Exanthems (<1%)
Exfoliative dermatitis (<1%)
Facial edema (<1%)
Furunculosis (<1%)
Herpes simplex (<1%)
Herpes zoster (<1%)
Lichenoid eruption (<1%)
Peripheral edema
Photosensitivity (<1%)
Pruritus (1–10%)
Psoriasis (<1%)
Pustules (<1%)
Rash (sic) (3%)
Urticaria (<1%)
Vesiculobullous eruption (<1%)
Xerosis (<1%)

Hair
Hair – alopecia (<1%) [1]
Hair – hirsutism (<1%)
Hair – pigmentation (<1%)

Hematopoietic
Ecchymoses (<1%)

Cardiovascular
Congestive heart failure [1]
QT prolongation [1]

Other
Ageusia (<1%)
Bromhidrosis (<1%)
Bruxism [1]
Dysgeusia (2%)
Galactorrhea [1]
Gingivitis (<1%)
Glossitis (<1%)
Gynecomastia (<1%)
Headache
Hyperesthesia (<1%)
Mastodynia [2]
Myalgia (>1%)
Oral ulceration (<1%)
Paresthesias (3%)
Parosmia (<1%)
Serotonin syndrome [5]
Sialorrhea (<1%)
Stomatitis (<1%)
Thrombophlebitis (<1%)
Tinnitus
Tongue edema (<1%)
Tongue pigmentation (<1%)
Tremor (1–10%)
Vaginitis
Vulvovaginal candidiasis (<1%)
Xerostomia (22%) [2]

VIGABATRIN

Trade name: Sabril (Ovation)
Indications: Epilepsy, infantile spasms (West's syndrome)
Category: Anticonvulsant; Antiepileptic
Half-life: 5-8 hours (young adults); 12-13 hours (elderly)
Clinically important, potentially hazardous interactions with: phenytoin

Reactions

Eyes
  Dyschromatopsia (blue-yellow)
  Eye pain

Other
  Abdominal pain (1.4%)
  Anxiety
  Asthenia (1.1%)
  Depression (2.5%) [2]
  Dizziness (3.8%)

Fatigue (9.2%)
Gingival hypertrophy [1]
Headache (3.8%) [1]
Joint pains
Paresthesias
Psychosis [3]
Seizures [2]
Sialorrhea
Tremor

ZALEPLON

Trade name: Sonata (Wyeth)
Indications: Insomnia
Category: Nonbenzodiazepine sedative-hypnotic
Half-life: 1 hour

Reactions

Skin
  Acne (<1%)
  Cheilitis (<1%)
  Chills (<1%)
  Dermatitis (<1%)
  Diaphoresis (<1%)
  Eczema (<1%)
  Edema (<1%)
  Exanthems (<1%)
  Facial edema (<1%)
  Peripheral edema (1–10%)
  Photosensitivity (1–10%)
  Pigmentation (<1%)
  Pruritus (<1%)
  Psoriasis (<1%)

Purpura (<1%)
Pustules (<1%)
Rash (sic) (<1%)
Vesiculobullous eruption (<1%)
Xerosis (<1%)

Hair
  Hair – alopecia (<1%)

Hematopoietic
  Ecchymoses (<1%)

Other
  Ageusia (<1%)
  Aphthous stomatitis (<1%)
  Gingival hemorrhage (<1%)
  Gingivitis (<1%)

Glossitis (<1%)
Headache
Hyperesthesia (<1%)
Mastodynia (<1%)
Myalgia (5%)
Oral ulceration (<1%)
Paresthesias (3%)
Parosmia (2%)

Sialorrhea (<1%)
Stomatitis (<1%)
Thrombophlebitis (<1%)
Tongue pigmentation (<1%)
Tremor (1–10%)
Vaginitis (<1%)
Xerostomia (1–10%)

ZIPRASIDONE

Synonym: Zeldox
Trade name: Geodon (Pfizer)
Indications: Schizophrenia
Category: Antipsychotic (benzothiazolylpiperazine); Serotonin & dopamine antagonist
Half-life: 4–5 hours
Clinically important, potentially hazardous interactions with: moxifloxacin, pimozide

Reactions

Skin
  Chills (<1%)
  Dermatitis
  Eczema (<1%)
  Exanthems (<1%)
  Exfoliative dermatitis (<1%)
  Facial edema (<1%)
  Fungal dermatitis (2%)
  Neuroleptic malignant syndrome [1]
  Peripheral edema (<1%)
  Photosensitivity (<1%)
  Rash (sic) (4%)
  Upper respiratory infection (8%)
  Urticaria (5%)
  Vesiculobullous eruption (<1%)

Hair
  Hair – alopecia (<1%)

Hematopoietic
  Ecchymoses (<1%)

Cardiovascular
  Arrhythmias [1]

Other
  Gingival hemorrhage (<1%)
  Gynecomastia (<1%)
  Headache
  Hyperesthesia (<1%)
  Myalgia (1%)
  Paresthesias (<1%)
  Priapism [2]
  Rhabdomyolysis [1]
  Sialorrhea
  Tardive dyskinesia [1]
  Thrombophlebitis (<1%)
  Tinnitus (<1%)
  Tongue edema (<1%)
  Tremor (<1%)
  Xerostomia (4%)

ZOLPIDEM

Trade name: Ambien (Sanofi-Aventis)
Other common trade names: *Niotal; Stilnoct; Stilnox*
Indications: Insomnia
Category: Nonbenzodiazepine sedative-hypnotic
Half-life: 2.6 hours
Clinically important, potentially hazardous interactions with: antihistamines, azatadine, azelastine, brompheniramine, buclizine, chlorpheniramine, clemastine, dexchlorpheniramine, meclizine, ritonavir

Reactions

Skin
Acne (<1%)
Allergic reactions (sic) (4%)
Bullous eruption (<1%)
Dermatitis (<1%)
Diaphoresis (<1%)
Edema (<1%)
Facial edema (<1%)
Furunculosis (<1%)
Herpes simplex (<1%)
Herpes zoster (<1%)
Photosensitivity (<1%)
Pruritus [1]
Purpura (<1%)
Rash (sic) (2%)
Urticaria (<1%)

Eyes
Periorbital edema (<1%)

Cardiovascular
Flushing (<1%)
Hot flashes (<1%)

Other
Anaphylactoid reactions (<1%)
Dysgeusia (<1%)
Hallucinations [2]
Headache
Hyperesthesia (<1%)
Injection-site inflammation (<1%)
Mastodynia (<1%)
Myalgia (7%)
Paresthesias (<1%)
Seizures [2]
Tinnitus
Tremor (<1%)
Vaginitis (<1%)
Xerostomia (3%)

ZONISAMIDE*

Trade name: Zonegran (Eisai)
Indications: Epilepsy
Category: Anticonvulsant sulfonamide
Half-life: 63 hours
Clinically important, potentially hazardous interactions with: caffeine

Reactions

Skin

Acne (<1%)
Allergic reactions (sic) (<1%)
Diaphoresis (<1%)
Eczema (<1%)
Edema (<1%)
Exanthems (<1%)
Facial edema (<1%)
Lupus erythematosus (<1%)
Peripheral edema (<1%)
Petechiae (<1%)
Pruritus (<1%)
Purpura (2%)
Pustules (<1%)
Rash (sic) (3%)
Stevens–Johnson syndrome [1]
Toxic epidermal necrolysis
Urticaria (<1%)
Vesiculobullous eruption (<1%)
Xerosis (<1%)

Hair

Hair – alopecia (<1%)
Hair – hirsutism (<1%)

Hematopoietic

Ecchymoses (2%)

Other

Dysgeusia (2%)
Gingival hypertrophy (<1%)
Gingivitis (<1%)
Glossitis (<1%)
Gynecomastia (<1%) [1]
Headache
Hyperesthesia (<1%)
Hyperpyrexia [1]
Hypersensitivity
Myalgia (<1%)
Oligohydrosis [4]
Oral ulceration (<1%)
Paresthesias (4%)
Parosmia (<1%)
Restless legs syndrome [1]
Stomatitis (<1%)
Thrombophlebitis (<1%)
Tremor (<1%) [1]
Ulcerative stomatitis (<1%)
Xerostomia (2%)

*Note: Zonisamide is a sulfonamide and can be absorbed systemically. Sulfonamides can produce severe, possibly fatal, reactions such as toxic epidermal necrolysis and Stevens–Johnson syndrome

DRUGS RESPONSIBLE FOR COMMON PSYCHIATRIC REACTIONS

ABNORMAL DREAMS
Acebutolol (2%)
Almotriptan
Alosetron
Alprazolam (2%)
Amantadine (1–5%)
Amlodipine
Aripiprazole
Atenolol
Atomoxetine
Bupropion
Cefditoren
Clomipramine
Clonidine
Codeine
Cyclobenzaprine
Donepezil
Efavirenz
Emtricitabine
Enflurane
Flecainide
Fluphenazine
Frovatriptan
Gatifloxacin
Glatiramer
Halothane
Hydrocodone
Isoflurane
Ketamine
Levofloxacin
Lomefloxacin
Mefloquine
Meperidine
Mesoridazine
Methadone
Methohexital
Methoxyflurane
Methyldopa
Mirtazapine
Montelukast
Morphine
Moxifloxacin
Nalbuphine
Nefazodone
Nicotine
Norfloxacin
Ofloxacin
Olanzapine
Oxycodone
Paroxetine
Pentazocine
Perphenazine
Pilocarpine
Pramipexole (>10%)
Prochlorperazine
Promazine
Promethazine
Propofol
Propoxyphene
Reserpine
Ropinirole
Secobarbital
Telithromycin
Verapamil
Zaleplon
Zolpidem

AGGRESSION
Acyclovir (<1%)
Azithromycin
Bupropion
Buspirone
Carbamazepine
Citalopram
Clonazepam
Daptomycin

Diethylpropion
Efavirenz
Ethosuximide
Felbamate
Fluoxetine
Flurazepam
Gabapentin
Galantamine
Isotretinoin
Lamotrigine
Levetiracetam
Mazindol
Mefloquine
Memantine
Methsuximide
Olanzapine (>10%)
Oxcarbazepine
Phendimetrazine
Phentermine
Rasburicase
Reteplase
Rifapentine
Risperidone
Rivastigmine
Streptokinase
Tiagabine
Topiramate
Urokinase
Vigabatrin
Ziprasidone

AKATHISIA

Albuterol
Almotriptan
Alprazolam (1.6–3%)
Amitriptyline
Amoxapine
Aripiprazole
Bendroflumethiazide
Benzphetamine
Bepridil
Buclizine
Carbamazepine
Chlordiazepoxide

Chlorothiazide
Chlorpromazine
Cinoxacin
Ciprofloxacin
Citalopram
Clemastine
Clomiphene
Clonidine
Clozapine
Cocaine
Codeine
Corticosteroids
Cyclobenzaprine
Cycloserine
Danazol
Desflurane
Desipramine
Dextroamphetamine
Dextromethorphan
Dicyclomine
Didanosine
Diethylpropion
Dihydroergotamine
Dimenhydrinate
Diphenoxylate
Dronabinol
Droperidol
Duloxetine
Entacapone
Ethchlorvynol
Ethionamide
Ethotoin
Fentanyl
Flavoxate
Fludarabine
Flumazenil
Fluoxetine
Fluphenazine
Fluvoxamine
Fluoxymesterone
Furosemide
Gabapentin
Glipizide
Glyburide

Glycopyrrolate
Guanabenz
Haloperidol
Hydrocodone
Hydroxychloroquine
Hydroxyurea
Imipramine
Indapamide
Isoetharine
Isoproterenol
Isosorbide dinitrate
Isosorbide mononitrate
Lindane
Lithium
Lorazepam
Loxapine
Maprotiline
Mazindol
Memantine
Meperidine
Mephenytoin
Mesoridazine
Metaxalone
Methadone
Methamphetamine
Methocarbamol
Metoclopramide
Molindone
Montelukast
Morphine
Nalbuphine
Nalidixic acid
Naloxone
Naltrexone
Nelfinavir
Nitroglycerin
Nortriptyline
Olanzapine
Olmesartan
Orphenadrine
Oxazepam
Oxcarbazepine
Oxybutynin
Oxycodone

Palonosetron
Paroxetine
Peginterferon alfa-2B
Pemoline
Pentazocine
Perphenazine
Phendimetrazine
Phentermine
Phenylephrine
Phenytoin
Physostigmine
Pirbuterol (>10%)
Pramipexole
Prazepam
Primidone
Prochlorperazine
Procyclidine
Promazine
Promethazine
Propoxyphene
Protriptyline
Pseudoephedrine
Quazepam
Rimantadine
Risperidone
Ritodrine
Sermorelin
Temazepam
Theophylline
Thioridazine
Thiothixene
Topiramate
Trazodone
Triazolam
Zonisamide

AMNESIA

Acamprosate
Alprazolam (10–33%)
Amantadine (<1%)
Amlodipine
Anagrelide
Aripiprazole
Atenolol

Benztropine
Bupropion
Carmustine
Chlordiazepoxide (>10%)
Cidofovir
Citalopram
Clomipramine
Clonidine
Clorazepate
Diazepam
Diltiazem
Doxazosin
Dronabinol
Efavirenz
Estazolam
Etodolac
Flecainide
Flurazepam
Flurbiprofen
Fluvastatin
Fluvoxamine
Fosphenytoin
Frovatriptan
Gabapentin
Interferon beta-1B
Labetalol
Lamotrigine
Leuprolide
Levetiracetam
Loratadine
Lorazepam
Lovastatin
Meclizine
Methocarbamol
Metoprolol
Midazolam
Miglustat
Modafinil
Nadolol
Naproxen
Nefazodone
Nifedipine
Olanzapine
Oxazepam

Oxcarbazepine
Penbutolol
Perindopril
Phenindamine
Pindolol
Piroxicam
Pramipexole
Pravastatin
Prazepam
Procyclidine
Propantheline
Propranolol
Quazepam
Rabeprazole
Ramipril
Ropinirole
Sodium oxybate
Tiagabine
Topiramate
Vigabatrin
Zalcitabine
Zaleplon
Ziprasidone
Zonisamide

ANOREXIA

Alemtuzumab (20%)
Anagrelide
Aprepitant
Calcitonin
Carbamazepine
Carboplatin
Caspofungin
Cefditoren
Cefuroxime
Celecoxib
Cetirizine
Ciprofloxacin
Citalopram
Clarithromycin
Colchicine
Cyclobenzaprine
Desipramine
Diphenhydramine

Donepezil
Doxepin
Efavirenz
Enalapril
Enfuvirtide
Ephedrine
Epinephrine
Epirubicin
Estramustine
Ethambutol
Etoposide
Famotidine
Fenofibrate
Fludarabine
Fluoxetine
Fluoxymesterone
Fluphenazine
Flurbiprofen
Flutamide
Fluvoxamine
Fondaparinux
Foscarnet
Fosphenytoin
Fulvestrant
Gabapentin
Galantamine
Ganciclovir (15%)
Gatifloxacin
Gefitinib
Gemcitabine
Gemtuzumab (31%)
Gentamicin
Glatiramer
Glimepiride
Glipizide
Glucagon
Gold
Goserelin
Haloperidol
Hyaluronic acid
Hydralazine
Hydrochlorothiazide
Hydrocodone
Hydroflumethiazide

Hydroxychloroquine
Hydroxyurea
Ibritumomab
Ibuprofen
Ifosfamide
Imatinib
Imipramine
Inamrinone
Indapamide
Indinavir
Indomethacin
Interferon alfa-2A (30–70%)
Irinotecan
Isoniazid
Itraconazole
Ivermectin
Ketamine
Ketoconazole
Ketoprofen
Lamivudine
Lamotrigine
Lansoprazole
Laronidase
Leflunomide
Letrozole
Leuprolide
Levalbuterol
Levetiracetam
Levodopa
Levofloxacin
Lithium
Lomefloxacin
Lomustine
Loracarbef
Loratadine
Lovastatin
Mechlorethamine
Meclizine
Meclofenamate
Mefenamic acid
Memantine
Meperidine
Mephenytoin
Mercaptopurine

Mesalamine
Mesoridazine
Metformin
Methadone
Methamphetamine
Methazolamide
Methohexital
Methotrexate
Methoxyflurane
Methyclothiazide
Methylphenidate
Methyltestosterone
Methysergide
Metoclopramide
Metronidazole
Miglustat
Mitomycin
Mitotane (24%)
Modafinil
Montelukast
Morphine
Moxifloxacin
Nalbuphine
Naltrexone
Naproxen
Natalizumab
Nefazodone
Nelfinavir
Niacin
Nicotine
Nitazoxanide
Nitisinone
Nitrofurantoin
Nizatidine
Norfloxacin
Nortriptyline
Octreotide
Ofloxacin
Olanzapine
Olmesartan
Olsalazine
Omeprazole
Oxaliplatin (20%)
Oxaprozin

Oxycodone
Palivizumab
Palonosetron
Pamidronate
Paramethadione
Paroxetine
Peginterferon alfa-2B
Pegvisomant
Pemetrexed (35–62%)
Pemoline
Penicillamine
Pentamidine
Pentazocine
Pentosan
Pentostatin (>10%)
Pergolide
Perphenazine
Phenindamine
Phenytoin
Pilocarpine
Pimecrolimus
Pimozide
Piroxicam
Plicamycin
Polythiazide
Pramipexole
Pravastatin
Praziquantel
Primaquine
Primidone
Probenecid
Procainamide
Prochlorperazine
Promazine
Promethazine
Propantheline
Propofol
Propoxyphene
Protriptyline
Pyrazinamide
Pyrimethamine
Quetiapine
Quinidine (>10%)
Raloxifene

Ranitidine
Reserpine
Ribavirin
Rifabutin
Rifampin
Rifapentine
Riluzole
Rimantadine
Risperidone
Ritodrine
Ritonavir
Rituximab
Rivastigmine (17%)
Ropinirole
Rosiglitazone
Rosuvastatin
Temozolomide
Venlafaxine

ANXIETY

Acamprosate (5%)
Acebutolol
Acitretin (<1%)
Acamprosate
Adenosine (1%)
Agalsidase (28%)
Aldesleukin (12%)
Almotriptan
Alosetron
Alprazolam (1–17%)
Amantadine (1–5%)
Amitriptyline
Amlodipine
Apomorphine
Amoxapine
Amoxicillin
Amphotericin B
Anastrozole
Aprepitant
Aripiprazole
Aprotinin
Arsenic
Atazanavir
Azacitidine

Azithromycin
Balsalazide
Basiliximab
Benazepril
Benzphetamine
Bepridil
Bicalutamide
Bismuth
Bivalirudin
Bortezomib (14%)
Botulinum toxin (a & b)
Bretylium
Bupropion
Calcitonin
Candesartan
Cefaclor
Cefpodoxime
Celecoxib
Cidofovir
Cimetidine
Citalopram
Clarithromycin
Clofarabine (22%)
Clomipramine
Clonazepam
Clopidogrel
Clorazepate
Clozapine
Colestipol
Corticosteroids
Cyanocobalamin
Cycloserine
Daclizumab
Daptomycin
Darbepoetin alfa
Desipramine
Dextroamphetamine
Diazepam
Dicloxacillin
Didanosine
Digoxin
Dihydroergotamine
Dimercaprol
Dinoprostone

Disopyramide
Donepezil
Dopamine
Droperidol
Doxazosin
Dronabinol (>10%)
Droperidol
Duloxetine
Efavirenz (1–11%)
Enfuvirtide
Enoxaparin
Entacapone
Ephedrine
Epinephrine
Epoetin alfa
Ertapenem
Escitalopram
Estazolam
Etanercept
Etodolac
Exemestane (10%)
Felbamate
Felodipine
Fenofibrate
Fentanyl
Flecainide
Flumazenil
Fluoxetine
Flurazepam
Flurbiprofen
Flutamide
Fomepizole
Foscarnet
Frovatriptan
Fulvestrant
Gabapentin
Gadodiamide
Gatifloxacin
Glatiramer (23%)
Glipizide
Goserelin
Guanabenz
Haloperidol
Hydralazine

Ibuprofen
Idebenone
Imipramine
Immune globulin IV
Indapamide
Indomethacin
Interferon beta-1A
Interferon beta-1B (10%)
Irbesartan
Isocarboxazid
Isradipine
Lamotrigine
Lansoprazole
Letrozole
Leuprolide
Levalbuterol
Levamisole
Levetiracetam
Levodopa
Levofloxacin
Levothyroxine
Lidocaine
Liothyronine
Lomefloxacin
Lovastatin
Mefloquine
Meloxicam
Metformin
Methamphetamine
Methicillin
Methyldopa
Methylphenidate
Metipranolol
Mezlocillin
Midodrine
Mifepristone
Mirtazapine
Misoprostol
Mitoxantrone
Modafinil
Molindone
Montelukast
Moxifloxacin
Mycophenolate (28%)

Nabumetone
Nafcillin
Naloxone
Naltrexone
Naproxen
Nateglinide
Nelfinavir
Nesiritide
Nicotine
Nisoldipine
Nitisinone
Norfloxacin
Nortriptyline
Octreotide
Ofloxacin
Olanzapine
Olsalazine
Ondansetron
Orlistat
Oxacillin
Oxaliplatin
Oxaprozin
Oxcarbazepine
Oxycodone
Palonosetron
Pantoprazole
Paroxetine
Peg-interferon alfa-2B (28%)
Penicillamine
Penicillins
Pentamidine
Pentazocine
Pentostatin
Pentoxifylline
Pergolide
Perindopril
Phenelzine
Phenobarbital
Phenylephrine
Pilocarpine
Pindolol
Piperacillin
Piroxicam
Pravastatin

Procyclidine
Propantheline
Propoxyphene
Protriptyline
Quetiapine
Quinidine
Quinine
Repaglinide
Reserpine
Rimantadine
Risperidone (>24%)
Ritodrine
Rituximab
Rivastigmine
Rizatriptan
Rosiglitazone
Rosuvastatin
Sibutramine
Sirolimus
Thiopental
Tizanidine
Tranylcypromine
Trimipramine
Venlafaxine
Vigabatrin
Zalcitabine
Zidovudine
Zolmitriptan
Zonisamide

APATHY
Alemtuzumab
Amlodipine
Aripiprazole
Benztropine
Bromocriptine
Citalopram
Digoxin
Flecainide
Levetiracetam
Zolpidem

APPETITE CHANGED
Carbamazepine

Cefditoren
Cefpodoxime
Celecoxib
Chlordiazepoxide (>10%)
Chlorotrianisene
Chlorpromazine
Citalopram
Cladribine
Clofibrate
Clomipramine (>10%)
Clorazepate
Codeine
Colchicine
Corticosteroids
Danazol
Dantrolene
Dapsone
Darbepoetin alfa
Demeclocycline
Denileukin
Dextroamphetamine
Dicumarol
Digoxin
Dihydrotachysterol
Diphenhydramine
Dofetilide
Doxazosin
Doxercalciferol
Dronabinol
Duloxetine (10%)
Efavirenz
Emtricitabine
Enflurane
Enfuvirtide
Eplerenone
Ergocalciferol
Escitalopram
Esomeprazole
Estrogens
Ethionamide
Ethotoin
Etodolac
Etoposide
Exemestane

Ezetimibe
Fenofibrate
Flecainide
Floxuridine
Fluconazole
Fluorouracil
Flutamide
Glimepiride
Halothane
Isoflurane
Leuprolide
Levothyroxine
Liothyronine
Maprotiline
Meclizine
Medroxyprogesterone
Mefloquine
Mirtazapine (17%)
Misoprostol
Nefazodone
Nicotine (>10%)
Nitazoxanide
Ofloxacin
Olanzapine
Paroxetine
Phytonadione
Quetiapine
Saquinavir
Secretin
Selegiline
Sertraline
Sibutramine
Sirolimus
Sodium oxybate
Somatropin
Stavudine
Streptokinase
Sulfadiazine
Sulfadoxine
Sulfamethoxazole
Sulfasalazine
Sulfinpyrazone
Tacrine
Tacrolimus

Telithromycin
Tenofovir
Terbinafine
Thiabendazole
Thioguanine
Thiotepa
Tiagabine
Ticlopidine
Tinidazole
Tinzaparin
Tiopronin
Tizanidine
Tocainide
Tolazamide
Tolbutamide
Topiramate
Topotecan
Toremifene
Tranylcypromine
Trazodone
Trimethadione
Trimetrexate
Trimipramine
Unoprostone
Urokinase
Vinorelbine
Voriconazole
Zafirlukast
Zidovudine
Ziprasidone
Zolmitriptan
Zonisamide

BEHAVIORAL CHANGES

Amoxicillin
Anastrozole
Biperiden
Clonazepam
Clonidine
Efavirenz
Fluoxetine
Flurazepam
Glycopyrrolate
Leuprolide

Olanzapine
Primidone
Rifampin
Zaleplon
Zolpidem

CATATONIA

Chlorpromazine
Citalopram
Labetalol
Metoprolol
Nadolol
Penbutolol
Pindolol
Propranolol

CHOREOATHETOSIS

Citalopram

COGNITIVE CHANGES

Abciximab (<1%)
Acamprosate
Aldesleukin (>10%)
Alemtuzumab
Alosetron
Alprazolam (29%)
Amitriptyline
Amphotericin B
Aripiprazole
Carvedilol
Ethosuximide
Flurazepam
Fluvoxamine
Gatifloxacin
Halothane
Imipenem/Cilastatin
Leuprolide
Levetiracetam
Levodopa
Levofloxacin
Lomefloxacin
Mirtazapine
Moxifloxacin
Norfloxacin

Oxycodone
Pentazocine
Pentobarbital
Propranolol
Phenobarbital
Propoxyphene
Zolpidem

CONCENTRATION IMPAIRED

Aripiprazole
Bupropion
Cabergoline
Carvedilol
Citalopram
Dicyclomine
Doxazosin
Efavirenz
Ethionamide
Ethosuximide
Fluoxetine
Frovatriptan
Gabapentin
Glycopyrrolate
Insulin
Lamotrigine
Loratadine
Metformin
Methsuximide
Nefazodone
Nicotine
Octreotide
Peginterferon alfa-2B (5–12%)
Pemetrexed
Phenindamine
Quinine
Reserpine
Ribavirin
Rimantadine
Sodium oxybate
Telithromycin
Tiagabine
Topiramate
Trazodone
Vigabatrin

Zalcitabine
Zonisamide

CONFUSION

Abciximab (<1%)
Acetazolamide
Adalimumab (<5%)
Aldesleukin (34%)
Alemtuzumab
Alosetron
Alprazolam(10%)
Amantadine (1–5%)
Amiloride
Amitriptyline
Amoxapine
Amoxicillin
Amphotericin B
Anagrelide
Anastrozole
Apomorphine
Aprepitant
Aprotinin
Aripiprazole
Arsenic
Asparaginase
Aspirin
Aztreonam
Baclofen
Benzonatate
Benztropine
Bexarotene
Bicalutamide
Bismuth
Bisoprolol
Bivalirudin
Bleomycin
Botulinum toxin (a & b)
Bupropion
Buspirone
Cabergoline
Capecitabine
Captopril
Carbamazepine (1–10%)
Carmustine (23%)

Carteolol
Cefaclor
Cefepime
Cefprozil
Cephalexin
Cetirizine
Cevimeline
Chloral hydrate
Chlorambucil
Chloramphenicol
Chlorotrianisene
Chlorthalidone
Cidofovir
Cimetidine
Ciprofloxacin
Citalopram
Clarithromycin
Clemastine
Clomipramine
Clonazepam
Clorazepate
Clozapine
Co-Trimoxazole
Cocaine
Codeine
Corticosteroids
Cyclobenzaprine
Cyclophosphamide
Cycloserine
Cyclosporine
Cytarabine
Dantrolene
Daptomycin
Darbepoetin alfa
Denileukin
Desipramine
Dextromethorphan
Diazepam
Diazoxide
Dicloxacillin
Dicumarol
Dicyclomine
Diethylpropion
Digoxin

Diphenhydramine
Disopyramide
Docetaxel
Docusate
Dofetilide
Doxazosin
Doxepin
Dronabinol (30%)
Efavirenz
Enoxaparin
Eplerenone
Ertapenem
Escitalopram
Esmolol
Esomeprazole
Estazolam
Etanercept
Ethacrynic acid
Ethambutol
Ethchlorvynol
Ethionamide
Ethotoin
Etodolac
Exemestane
Fentanyl
Flavoxate
Flecainide
Flucytosine
Fludarabine
Flumazenil
Fluoxetine
Fluoxymesterone
Fluphenazine
Flurazepam
Flurbiprofen
Flutamide
Fluvoxamine
Fondaparinux
Foscarnet
Fosinopril
Fosphenytoin
Frovatriptan
Gabapentin
Gadodiamide

Galantamine
Ganciclovir
Gatifloxacin
Gemtuzumab
Glatiramer
Glimepiride
Glipizide
Glyburide
Glycopyrrolate
Gold
Griseofulvin
Guanfacine
Haloperidol
Hydrochlorothiazide
Hydrocodone
Hydroflumethiazide
Hydroxyurea
Hyoscyamine
Ibandronate
Ibritumomab
Ibuprofen
Ifosfamide
Imipenem/Cilastatin
Imipramine
Immune globulin IV
Indinavir
Indomethacin
Insulin
Interferon alfa-2A
Interferon beta-1A
Interferon beta-1B
Irbesartan
Isocarboxazid
Ketoprofen
Labetalol
Lamotrigine
Laronidase
Leflunomide
Letrozole
Leuprolide
Levamisole
Levetiracetam
Levodopa
Levofloxacin

Lithium
Lomefloxacin
Lomustine
Loratadine
Lorazepam
Loxapine
Maprotiline
Mazindol
Mecamylamine
Meclofenamate
Mefenamic acid
Mefloquine
Meloxicam
Memantine
Mepenzolate
Meperidine
Mephenytoin
Mephobarbital
Meprobamate
Mesoridazine
Metaxalone
Metformin
Methadone
Methantheline
Methazolamide
Methicillin
Methocarbamol
Methotrexate
Methyclothiazide
Methyltestosterone
Metoclopramide
Metoprolol
Metronidazole
Mexiletine
Mezlocillin
Midodrine
Mirtazapine
Misoprostol
Mitotane
Modafinil
Molindone
Morphine (>10%)
Moxifloxacin
Mycophenolate

Nabumetone
Nadolol
Nafcillin
Nalbuphine
Nalidixic acid
Naltrexone
Naproxen
Naratriptan
Natalizumab
Nateglinide
Nefazodone
Nesiritide
Nicotine
Nisoldipine
Nitisinone
Nizatidine
Norfloxacin
Nortriptyline
Octreotide
Ofloxacin
Olmesartan
Orphenadrine
Oseltamivir
Oxacillin
Oxaprozin
Oxazepam
Oxcarbazepine
Oxybutynin
Oxycodone
Palonosetron
Pamidronate
Pantoprazole
Paramethadione
Paroxetine
Pegaptanib
Pemetrexed
Pemoline
Penbutolol
Penicillins
Pentazocine
Pentobarbital
Pentostatin
Pentoxifylline
Pergolide (10%)

Perphenazine
Phenazopyridine
Phendimetrazine
Phenelzine
Phenindamine
Phenobarbital
Phenoxybenzamine
Phentermine
Phenytoin
Pilocarpine
Pindolol
Piperacillin
Piroxicam
Polythiazide
Potassium iodide
Pramipexole
Prazepam
Primidone
Procainamide
Procarbazine (>10%)
Prochlorperazine
Procyclidine
Promazine
Promethazine
Propantheline
Propoxyphene
Propranolol
Protriptyline
Quazepam
Quinidine
Quinine
Ranitidine
Rasburicase
Repaglinide
Reteplase
Rifampin
Rimantadine
Ritonavir
Rivastigmine
Rizatriptan
Ropinirole
Rosiglitazone
Salsalate
Selegiline

Sirolimus
Sodium oxybate
Sparfloxacin
Spironolactone
Streptokinase
Streptozocin
Sufentanil
Tegaserod
Telithromycin
Thiabendazole
Thiopental
Tiagabine
Tinzaparin
Tocainide
Tolazamide
Tolbutamide
Tolcapone
Topiramate
Toremifene
Travoprost
Trazodone
Trihexyphenidyl
Treprostinil
Trimetrexate
Trimipramine
Urokinase
Valacyclovir
Valganciclovir
Vasopressin
Vigabatrin
Voriconazole
Zalcitabine
Zaleplon
Zidovudine
Ziprasidone
Zoledronic acid
Zolpidem

CHRONIC FATIGUE SYNDROME
Anthrax vaccine
Fluorides

DELIRIUM
Acyclovir (<1%)

Amantadine
Amphotericin B
Aripiprazole
Cevimeline
Chloramphenicol
Chloroquine
Ciprofloxacin
Desipramine
Dicyclomine
Digoxin
Galantamine
Glycopyrrolate
Imipramine
Interferon alfa-2A
Interferon beta-1B
Nortriptyline
Oxcarbazepine
Propofol
Protriptyline
Quinidine
Rabeprazole
Rivastigmine
Ziprasidone

DELUSIONS
Aripiprazole
Citalopram
Clonazepam
Donepezil
Dronabinol
Efavirenz
Felbamate
Flurazepam
Gabapentin
Imipramine
Losartan
Methylphenidate
Nortriptyline
Protriptyline
Ritonavir
Trihexyphenidyl
Zonisamide

DEMENTIA
Gabapentin
Leuprolide
Ritonavir
Zalcitabine

DEPERSONALIZATION
Alprazolam (1–10%)
Amlodipine
Aripiprazole
Bupropion
Cevimeline
Chloroquine
Ciprofloxacin
Citalopram
Clarithromycin
Clomipramine
Dextroamphetamine
Dipyridamole
Doxazosin
Dronabinol
Flecainide
Flumazenil
Fluoxymesterone
Frovatriptan
Gatifloxacin
Interferon beta-1B
Lamotrigine
Levetiracetam
Levofloxacin
Lomefloxacin
Methamphetamine
Methyltestosterone
Moxifloxacin
Norfloxacin
Ofloxacin
Ribavirin
Sodium oxybate
Topiramate
Zalcitabine

DEPRESSION
Acamprosate (4%)
Acebutolol (2%)

Acetazolamide
Acitretin (1–10%)
Acyclovir (<1%)
Acamprosate
Agalsidase (10%)
Aldesleukin
Alemtuzumab (7%)
Alfentanil (1–10%)
Almotriptan
Alosetron
Alprazolam (14%)
Altretamine (<1%)
Amantadine (1–5%)
Amiloride
Amitriptyline
Amlodipine
Amphotericin B
Amprenavir
Anagrelide
Anastrozole
Anthrax vaccine
Apomorphine
Apraclonidine
Aprepitant
Aripiprazole
Arsenic
Asparaginase
Atazanavir
Atenolol
Atomoxetine
Azacitidine
Baclofen
Balsalazide
Basiliximab
Benzphetamine
Benztropine
Bepridil
Bexarotene
Betaxolol
Bicalutamide
Bismuth
Bisoprolol
Botulinum toxin (a & b)
Brimonidine

Bromocriptine
Bupropion
Cabergoline
Caffeine
Calcitonin
Candesartan
Capecitabine
Captopril
Carbamazepine
Carisoprodol
Carmustine (16%)
Carteolol
Carvedilol
Celecoxib
Cetuximab
Cevimeline
Chloramphenicol
Chloroquine
Chlorotrianisene
Cimetidine
Ciprofloxacin
Citalopram
Clofarabine (11%)
Clofazimine
Clomiphene
Clonazepam
Clonidine
Clopidogrel
Clorazepate
Clozapine
Co-Trimoxazole
Codeine
Corticosteroids
Cyclobenzaprine
Cycloserine
Cyproheptadine
Dacarbazine
Dantrolene
Daptomycin
Dextroamphetamine
Diazepam
Dicloxacillin
Dicyclomine
Diethylpropion

Digoxin
Diltiazem
Diphenoxylate
Disopyramide
Domperidone
Donepezil
Doxazosin
Doxorubicin
Dronabinol
Efavirenz (1–16%)
Eletriptan
Emtricitabine (10%)
Enalapril
Enfuvirtide
Eprosartan
Ertapenem
Escitalopram
Esmolol
Esomeprazole
Estazolam
Estrogens
Etanercept
Ethionamide
Ethosuximide
Etodolac
Exemestane (13%)
Felbamate
Felodipine
Fenofibrate
Fenoprofen
Fentanyl
Finasteride
Flecainide
Floxuridine
Flumazenil
Fluoxetine
Fluoxymesterone
Fluphenazine
Flurazepam
Flurbiprofen
Flutamide
Fluvastatin
Fluvoxamine
Fosamprenavir

Foscarnet
Frovatriptan
Fulvestrant
Gabapentin
Galantamine
Gatifloxacin
Gemfibrozil
Gemtuzumab (10%)
Glatiramer
Glipizide
Glucosamine
Glycopyrrolate
Goldenseal
Goserelin (5–54%)
Granulocyte colony-stimulating factor (GCSF)
Guanfacine
Haloperidol
Horse chestnut (bark, flower, leaf, seed)
Hyaluronic acid
Hydralazine
Hydrochlorothiazide
Hydrocodone
Hydroflumethiazide
Ibuprofen
Imatinib
Imiquimod
Indapamide
Indinavir
Indomethacin
Infliximab
Interferon alfa-2A (>15%)
Interferon beta-1A (20%)
Interferon beta-1B
Irbesartan
Isoniazid
Isotretinoin
Isradipine
Ketoconazole
Ketoprofen
Lamivudine
Lamotrigine
Lansoprazole
Letrozole

Leuprolide
Levamisole
Levetiracetam
Levobetaxolol
Levobunolol
Levodopa
Levofloxacin
Lithium
Lomefloxacin
Loratadine
Lorazepam
Lovastatin
Mazindol
MDMA (37%)
Mecamylamine
Meclofenamate
Medroxyprogesterone
Mefenamic acid
Mefloquine
Meloxicam
Memantine
Meperidine
Mephenytoin
Mephobarbital
Mesoridazine
Metaxalone
Methadone
Methamphetamine
Methazolamide
Methicillin
Methimazole
Methoxsalen
Methsuximide
Methyclothiazide
Methyldopa
Methylphenidate
Methyltestosterone
Methysergide
Metipranolol
Metoclopramide
Metolazone
Metoprolol
Mexiletine
Mezlocillin

Misoprostol
Mitotane (32%)
Mitoxantrone
Modafinil
Molindone
Morphine
Moxifloxacin
Mycophenolate
Nabumetone
Nadolol
Nafarelin
Nafcillin
Nalbuphine
Naltrexone
Naproxen
Natalizumab
Nelfinavir
Niacin
Nifedipine
Nimodipine
Nitrofurantoin
Norfloxacin
Ofloxacin
Olsalazine
Oral contraceptives
Oxacillin
Oxaliplatin
Oxazepam
Oxaprozin
Oxycodone
Pantoprazole
Paroxetine
Peginterferon alfa-2B (16-29%)
Pemetrexed (11-14%)
Pemoline
Penbutolol
Pentazocine
Pentobarbital
Pentostatin
Pentoxifylline
Perindopril
Perphenazine
Phendimetrazine
Phenindamine

Phenobarbital
Phentermine
Phenylpropanolamine
Phenytoin
Pimozide
Pindolol
Piperacillin
Piroxicam
Plicamycin
Polythiazide
Pravastatin
Prazepam
Prazosin
Procainamide
Procarbazine (>10%)
Prochlorperazine
Progestins
Promazine
Promethazine
Propantheline
Propoxyphene
Propranolol
Pyrimethamine
Quazepam
Quinapril
Quinidine
Rabeprazole
Raloxifene
Ramipril
Rasburicase
Reserpine
Reteplase
Ribavirin
Riluzole
Risperidone
Rituximab
Rivastigmine
Rizatriptan
Ropinirole
Rosiglitazone
Rosuvastatin
Secobarbital
Sibutramine
Sirolimus

Sodium oxybate
Solifenacin
Streptokinase
Tamoxifen
Tartrazine
Tea tree
Tegaserod
Terbinafine
Teriparatide
Tiagabine
Timolol
Tinidazole
Tiotropium
Tizanidine
Topiramate
Trastuzumab
Travoprost
Tretinoin
Trihexyphenidyl
Trioxsalen
Triptorelin
Trovafloxacin
Urokinase
Ursodiol
Valdecoxib
Valsartan
Vigabatrin
Vinblastine
Voriconazole
Zalcitabine
Zaleplon
Zidovudine
Zolmitriptan
Zolpidem
Zonisamide

DISINHIBITION
Alprazolam (1–10%)
Chlordiazepoxide (1–10%)
Clonazepam

DISORIENTATION
Aldesleukin (>10%)
Amitriptyline

Amoxapine
Benztropine
Biperiden
Chloral hydrate
Cimetidine
Clarithromycin
Clonazepam
Desipramine
Domperidone
Doxepin
Ertapenem
Ethambutol
Flurazepam
Hydralazine
Hydroxyurea
Imipramine
Lorazepam
Methadone
Morphine
Nalbuphine
Naltrexone
Nortriptyline
Oxazepam
Oxcarbazepine
Pentazocine
Prazepam
Procainamide
Procarbazine (>10%)
Propoxyphene
Protriptyline
Quazepam

DIZZINESS
Abarelix (12%)
Acamprosate (3%)
Acebutolol (6%)
Acetazolamide
Acetohexamide
Acetylcysteine
Acitretin (<1%)
Acyclovir (1–10%)
Adenosine (1–10%)
Agalsidase (14%)
Albendazole (1–10%)

Albuterol
Aldesleukin (11%)
Alefacept (1–10%)
Alfuzosin (6%)
Almotriptan (>1%)
Alemtuzumab (12%)
Alprazolam (2–30%)
Alprostadil (2–10%)
Altretamine (<1%)
Amantadine (5–10%)
Amifostine
Amiloride
Aminocaproic acid
Aminophylline
Amiodarone
Amitriptyline
Amlodipine
Amoxapine
Amoxicillin
Amphotericin B
Anastrozole
Anthrax vaccine
Apomorphine
Apraclonidine
Aprepitant
Aprotinin
Aripiprazole
Arsenic
Ascorbic acid
Aspirin
Atazanavir
Atenolol
Atomoxetine
Azacitidine
Azithromycin
Aztreonam
Baclofen
Balsalazide
Basiliximab
Benazepril
Bendroflumethiazide
Benzonatate
Benzphetamine
Benztropine

Bepridil
Betaxolol
Bevacizumab
Bexarotene
Bicalutamide
Black cohosh
Bortezomib (21%)
Botulinum toxin (a & b)
Bretylium
Brinzolamide
Bromocriptine (17%)
Bumetanide
Bupropion
Buspirone (12%)
Cabergoline (17%)
Calcitonin
Carbinoxamine
Candesartan
Capecitabine
Capreomycin
Carbamazepine (>10%)
Carbinoxamine
Carisoprodol
Carmustine
Carteolol
Carvedilol (32%)
Cascara
Caspofungin
Cefaclor
Cefdinir
Cefditoren
Cefixime
Ceftazidime
Ceftibuten
Ceftriaxone
Cefuroxime
Celecoxib
Cephalexin
Cephradine
Cetirizine
Cevimeline
Chloral hydrate
Chlordiazepoxide (1–10%)
Chlorothiazide

Chlorotrianisene
Chlorpromazine
Chlorpropamide
Chlorthalidone
Chlorzoxazone
Cilostazol (10%)
Cimetidine
Cinacalcet (10%)
Cinoxacin
Ciprofloxacin
Citalopram
Cladribine
Clarithromycin
Clemastine
Clofarabine (16%)
Clofazimine
Clomiphene
Clomipramine (>10%)
Clonazepam (>10%)
Clonidine (16%)
Clopidogrel
Clorazepate
Clozapine (>10%)
Cocaine
Codeine
Colestipol
Corticosteroids
Cyanocobalamin
Cyclobenzaprine (11%)
Cyclophosphamide
Cycloserine
Cyproheptadine
Cytarabine
Dacarbazine
Daclizumab
Dalteparin
Danaparoid
Dantrolene
Daptomycin
Darbepoetin alfa
Delavirdine
Denileukin (22%)
Desflurane
Desipramine

Desloratadine
Desmopressin
Dextroamphetamine
Dextromethorphan
Diazepam
Diclofenac
Dicloxacillin
Dicumarol
Dicyclomine
Diethylpropion
Diflunisal
Digoxin
Dihydroergotamine
Diltiazem
Dimenhydrinate
Dinoprostone
Diphenhydramine
Diphenoxylate
Dipyridamole (14%)
Dirithromycin
Disopyramide
Dobutamine
Docetaxel
Docusate
Dofetilide
Dolasetron
Domperidone
Donepezil
Dorzolamide
Doxazosin (>16–19%)
Doxepin
Doxercalciferol (12%)
Doxorubicin
Doxycycline
Dronabinol (21%)
Duloxetine (10%)
Dutasteride
Echinacea
Edrophonium
Efavirenz (2–28%)
Eflornithine
Eletriptan
Emtricitabine (25%)
Enalapril

Enflurane
Enfuvirtide
Enoxaparin
Entacapone
Ephedrine
Epinephrine
Eplerenone
Epoetin alfa
Eprosartan
Ertapenem
Escitalopram
Esmolol
Esomeprazole
Estazolam
Estrogens
Etanercept
Ethacrynic acid
Ethambutol
Ethchlorvynol
Ethionamide
Ethosuximide
Ethotoin
Etodolac
Eucalyptus
Exemestane
Ezetimibe
Famciclovir
Famotidine
Felbamate
Felodipine
Fenofibrate
Fenoldopam
Fenoprofen (7–15%)
Fentanyl
Fexofenadine
Finasteride
Flavoxate
Flecainide (19%)
Floxuridine
Fluconazole
Flucytosine
Fludarabine
Flumazenil
Fluoxetine

Fluoxymesterone
Flurazepam
Flurbiprofen
Flutamide
Fluvastatin
Fluvoxamine
Fomepizole
Fondaparinux
Formoterol
Foscarnet
Fosfomycin
Fosinopril (2–12%)
Fosphenytoin (<10%)
Frovatriptan
Fulvestrant
Furosemide
Gabapentin (17%)
Gadodiamide
Galantamine
Gatifloxacin
Gemcitabine
Gemfibrozil
Gemifloxacin
Gemtuzumab (11%)
Gentamicin
Glatiramer
Glimepiride
Glipizide
Glucagon
Glyburide
Glycopyrrolate
Goserelin
Granisetron
Granulocyte colony-stimulating factor
(GCSF)
Griseofulvin
Guanabenz
Guanadrel
Guanethidine
Guanfacine
Guarana
Haloperidol
Halothane
Hawthorn (fruit, leaf, flower extract)

Heparin
Hepatitis B vaccine
Hyaluronic acid
Hydralazine
Hydrochlorothiazide
Hydrocodone
Hydroflumethiazide
Hydromorphone
Hydroxychloroquine
Hydroxyurea
Hyoscyamine
Ibandronate
Ibritumomab
Imiglucerase
Imipenem/Cilastatin
Imipramine
Imiquimod
Immune globulin IV
Inamrinone
Indapamide
Indinavir
Indomethacin
Infliximab
Influenza vaccines
Interferon alfa-2A (21%)
Interferon beta-1A (15%)
Interferon beta-1B (24%)
Ipodate
Ipratropium
Irbesartan (10%)
Irinotecan (10%)
Isocarboxazid
Isoetharine
Isoflurane
Isoniazid
Isosorbide dinitrate
Isosorbide mononitrate
Isotretinoin
Isoxsuprine
Isradipine
Itraconazole
Ivermectin
Kava
Ketamine

Ketoconazole
Ketoprofen
Ketorolac
Labetalol (<16%)
Lamivudine
Lamotrigine (38%)
Lansoprazole
Laronidase
Leflunomide
Letrozole
Levalbuterol
Levamisole
Levetiracetam (9–18%)
Levobetaxolol
Levobunolol
Levodopa
Levofloxacin
Lidocaine
Lindane
Linezolid
Lisinopril
Lithium
Lomefloxacin
Loperamide
Loracarbef
Loratadine
Lorazepam
Losartan
Lovastatin
Loxapine
Maprotiline
Mazindol
Mebendazole
Mecamylamine
Mechlorethamine
Meclizine
Meclofenamate
Medroxyprogesterone
Mefenamic acid
Mefloquine
Meloxicam
Memantine
Mepenzolate
Meperidine

Mephenytoin (<10%)
Mephobarbital
Meprobamate
Mesalamine
Metaxalone
Metformin
Methadone
Methamphetamine
Methantheline
Methazolamide
Methicillin
Methimazole
Methocarbamol
Methohexital
Methotrexate
Methoxsalen
Methoxyflurane
Methsuximide
Methyclothiazide
Methyldopa
Methylphenidate
Methyltestosterone
Methysergide
Metipranolol
Metolazone (>10%)
Metoprolol
Metronidazole
Mexiletine (20–25%)
Mezlocillin
Midodrine
Mifepristone (<12%)
Miglustat (<11%)
Minocycline
Mirtazapine
Mitotane (15%)
Modafinil
Molindone
Montelukast
Moricizine (>10%)
Morphine
Moxifloxacin
Mupirocin
Mycophenolate
Nabumetone (>10%)

Nadolol (<16%)
Nafcillin
Nalbuphine
Nalidixic acid
Naltrexone
Naproxen
Naratriptan
Natalizumab
Nateglinide
Nedocromil
Nefazodone (>10%)
Nelfinavir
Nesiritide
Nicardipine
Nicotine
Nifedipine (10–27%)
Nisoldipine
Nitazoxanide
Nitisinone
Nitrofurantoin
Nitroglycerin
Nizatidine
Norfloxacin
Nortriptyline
Octreotide
Ofloxacin
Olanzapine (>10%)
Olmesartan
Olsalazine
Omalizumab
Omeprazole
Ondansetron
Orphenadrine
Oxacillin
Oxaliplatin
Oxaprozin
Oxazepam
Oxcarbazepine (22–44%)
Oxybutynin (6–16%)
Oxycodone (>10%)
Oxytetracycline
Paclitaxel
Palonosetron
Pamidronate

Pantoprazole
Papaverine
Paramethadione
Paricalcitol
Paromomycin
Paroxetine (>10%)
Peginterferon alfa-2B (12%)
Pegaptanib
Pegvisomant
Pemetrexed
Pemoline
Penbutolol (<16%)
Penicillins
Pentagastrin
Pentazocine
Pentobarbital
Pentosan
Pentostatin
Pentoxifylline
Perflutren
Pergolide (19%)
Perindopril
Perphenazine
Phenazopyridine
Phendimetrazine
Phenelzine
Phenindamine
Phenobarbital
Phenoxybenzamine
Phentermine
Phentolamine
Phenylephrine
Phenytoin
Phytonadione
Pilocarpine
Pimozide
Pindolol
Piperacillin
Pirbuterol
Piroxicam (>10%)
Polythiazide
Pramipexole (>10%)
Pravastatin
Prazepam

Praziquantel
Prazosin (>10%)
Primaquine
Primidone
Probenecid
Procainamide
Procarbazine (>10%)
Prochlorperazine
Procyclidine
Progestins
Promazine
Promethazine
Propantheline (4–15%)
Propofol
Propoxyphene
Propranolol (<16%)
Propylthiouracil
Protriptyline
Pseudoephedrine
Pyrimethamine
Quazepam
Quetiapine (>10%)
Quinapril
Quinethazone
Quinidine (>15%)
Quinine
Rabeprazole
Ramipril
Ranitidine
Rasburicase
Reserpine
Reteplase
Ribavirin
Rifampin
Rifapentine
Rifaximin
Riluzole
Rimantadine
Risedronate
Risperidone (>19%)
Ritodrine
Ritonavir
Rituximab (>10%)
Rivastigmine (21%)

Rizatriptan
Rofecoxib
Ropinirole (40%)
Rosuvastatin
Salmeterol
Salsalate
Sargramostin
Scopolamine
Secretin
Selegiline
Sermorelin
Sertraline
Sibutramine
Sildenafil
Simvastatin
Sirolimus
Sodium oxybate
Solifenacin
Sotalol
Sparfloxacin
Spectinomycin
Spironolactone
St John's wort
Stavudine
Streptokinase
Streptomycin
Succimer
Sulfadiazine
Sulfamethoxazole
Sulindac
Sumatriptan
Tadalafil
Tamsulosin
Tegaserod
Telithromycin
Telmisartan
Temazepam
Tenecteplase
Terazosin
Terbutaline
Teriparatide
Thalidomide
Thiabendazole
Thioguanine

Thiopental
Thioridazine
Thiotepa
Thiothixene
Tiagabine
Ticarcillin
Timolol
Tinidazole
Tinzaparin
Tizanidine
Tocainide
Tolazamide
Tolbutamide
Tolcapone
Tolmetin
Topiramate
Toremifene
Torsemide
Tositumomab & iodine 131
Tramadol
Trandolapril
Travoprost
Trazodone
Treprostinil
Triamterene
Triazolam
Trichlormethiazide
Trifluoperazine
Trihexyphenidyl
Trimeprazine
Trimethobenzamide
Trimetrexate
Trimipramine
Trioxsalen
Tripelennamine
Triptorelin
Trovafloxacin
Ursodiol
Valdecoxib
Valrubicin
Valsartan
Vardenafil
Vasopressin
Venlafaxine

Verapamil
Vigabatrin
Vinblastine
Voriconazole
Zafirlukast
Zalcitabine
Zaleplon
Zanamivir
Zidovudine
Zileuton
Ziprasidone
Zoledronic acid
Zolmitriptan
Zonisamide

DYSARTHRIA

Acyclovir
Alprazolam (10–23%)
Aripiprazole
Baclofen
Capecitabine
Carbamazepine
Carmustine (11%)
Chlordiazepoxide (>10%)
Clomipramine
Clonazepam
Clonidine
Clorazepate
Clozapine
Cocaine
Cytarabine
Dantrolene
Denileukin
Diazepam
Dicyclomine
Diethylstilbestrol
Dofetilide
Donepezil
Doxazosin
Edrophonium
Efavirenz
Epoetin alfa
Estazolam
Estrogens

Ethchlorvynol
Ethotoin
Felbamate
Fluoxetine
Flurazepam
Fosphenytoin
Frovatriptan
Fulvestrant
Gabapentin
Gemcitabine
Glimepiride
Glipizide
Glyburide
Glycopyrrolate
Hyoscyamine
Imatinib
Immune globulin IV
Insulin
Irinotecan
Isocarboxazid
Isoniazid
Lamotrigine
Lidocaine
Lithium
Lomustine
Loxapine
Mephenytoin
Meprobamate
Mesoridazine
Metformin
Methantheline
Nateglinide
Olanzapine
Oxazepam
Perphenazine
Phenelzine
Phenytoin
Prazepam
Prochlorperazine
Promazine
Promethazine
Quetiapine
Rasburicase
Repaglinide

Rosiglitazone
Sirolimus
Sodium cromoglycate
Ziprasidone

Quazepam
Tizanidine
Zalcitabine
Zidovudine

EUPHORIA

Amantadine (<1%)
Aripiprazole
Baclofen
Biperiden
Citalopram
Clomipramine
Cocaine
Corticosteroids
Dextroamphetamine
Diphenhydramine
Felbamate
Flecainide
Flumazenil
Fluoxetine
Fluoxymesterone
Frovatriptan
Gatifloxacin
Haloperidol
Levofloxacin
Lomefloxacin
Meprobamate
Methadone
Methamphetamine
Methyltestosterone
Midazolam
Molindone
Morphine
Moxifloxacin
Nalbuphine
Norfloxacin
Ofloxacin
Olanzapine
Oxazepam
Oxycodone
Pentazocine
Phentermine
Prazepam
Propoxyphene

EXCITEMENT

Acetazolamide
Amoxapine
Baclofen
Buclizine
Buspirone
Carbinoxamine
Ceftazidime
Chloral hydrate
Chlordiazepoxide
Clonazepam
Clozapine
Cocaine
Codeine
Corticosteroids
Dextromethorphan
Diethylpropion
Diphenhydramine
Efavirenz
Ethchlorvynol
Ethotoin
Flavoxate
Fluoxetine
Fluphenazine
Glycopyrrolate
Hydrocodone
Hydroxychloroquine
Hydroxyurea
Isocarboxazid
Lithium
Maprotiline
Mazindol
Mecamylamine
Meperidine
Mephobarbital
Meprobamate
Mesoridazine
Methadone
Methysergide

Mirtazapine
Morphine
Nalbuphine
Nefazodone
Orphenadrine
Oxazepam
Oxybutynin
Oxycodone
Pentazocine
Pentobarbital
Pentoxifylline
Perphenazine
Phendimetrazine
Phenelzine
Phenobarbital
Phentermine
Phenylephrine
Prazepam
Primidone
Prochlorperazine
Procyclidine
Promazine
Promethazine
Propoxyphene
Pseudoephedrine
Quazepam
Risperidone
Salmeterol
Secobarbital
Sertraline
Tranylcypromine
Trimeprazine
Trimipramine
Triprolidine

HALLUCINATIONS

Acyclovir (<1%)
Alemtuzumab
Alendronate
Amantadine (1–5%)
Amitriptyline
Amphotericin B
Apomorphine
Aripiprazole

Asparaginase
Baclofen
Benzonatate
Benztropine
Bisoprolol
Bromocriptine
Buclizine
Bupropion
Caffeine
Carbamazepine
Carbinoxamine
Carteolol
Cefepime
Cephalexin
Cetirizine
Cevimeline
Chloral hydrate
Chlorambucil
Cimetidine
Ciprofloxacin
Citalopram
Clonazepam
Clonidine
Clozapine
Co-Trimoxazole
Cocaine
Codeine
Corticosteroids
Cyclobenzaprine
Delavirdine
Desipramine
Dicyclomine
Diethylpropion
Diflunisal
Digoxin
Dimenhydrinate
Dronabinol
Efavirenz
Enalapril
Entacapone
Ertapenem
Ethambutol
Etidronate
Etodolac

Felbamate
Flavoxate
Flucytosine
Fluoxetine
Flurazepam
Flurbiprofen
Gatifloxacin
Glatiramer
Glycopyrrolate
Gold
Goldenseal
Guanfacine
Haloperidol
Hydrocodone
Hydroxyurea
Hydroxyzine
Ibuprofen
Ifosfamide
Imipenem/Cilastatin
Imipramine
Indomethacin
Interferon alfa-2A
Interferon beta-1B
Isocarboxazid
Ketoprofen
Ketorolac
Levodopa
Levofloxacin
Lidocaine
Lomefloxacin
Maprotiline
Mazindol
Meclofenamate
Mefenamic acid
Mefloquine
Memantine
Meperidine
Mephobarbital
Methadone
Methysergide
Metoprolol
Mexiletine
Midazolam
Mirtazapine

Montelukast
Morphine
Mycophenolate
Moxifloxacin
Nadolol
Nalbuphine
Nalidixic acid
Naltrexone
Naproxen
Naratriptan
Nefazodone
Norfloxacin
Nortriptyline
Ofloxacin
Omeprazole
Orphenadrine
Oxybutynin
Oxycodone
Pamidronate
Peginterferon alfa-2B
Pemoline
Penbutolol
Pentazocine
Pentobarbital
Pentoxifylline
Pergolide (14%)
Phendimetrazine
Phenelzine
Phenobarbital
Phentermine
Physostigmine
Pindolol
Piroxicam
Pramipexole (>10%)
Prazosin
Procainamide
Procarbazine (>10%)
Procyclidine
Propoxyphene
Propranolol
Protriptyline
Pseudoephedrine
Quinidine
Ranitidine

Rimantadine
Risperidone
Ritonavir
Rivastigmine
Ropinirole
Sertraline
Sparfloxacin
Sufentanil
Thiabendazole
Thiopental
Tizanidine
Tolcapone
Tolterodine
Trihexyphenidyl
Trimipramine
Triprolidine
Trovafloxacin
Valganciclovir
Zalcitabine
Zaleplon
Zolpidem
Zonisamide

HYPERACTIVITY

Amoxapine
Amoxicillin
Aripiprazole
Cefpodoxime
Cefprozil
Fluvoxamine
Prochlorperazine
Promazine
Promethazine
Tartrazine
Vigabatrin

INSOMNIA

Abacavir (7%)
Acamprosate (6%)
Acebutolol (3%)
Acitretin (1–10%)
Acamprosate
Albuterol
Alemtuzumab (10%)

Almotriptan
Alprazolam (9–30%)
Amantadine (5–10%)
Amiloride
Aminophylline
Amiodarone
Amitriptyline
Amlodipine
Amoxapine
Amoxicillin
Amphotericin B
Anagrelide
Anastrozole
Apomorphine
Aprepitant
Aprotinin
Aripiprazole
Arsenic
Atazanavir
Atomoxetine
Aztreonam
Baclofen
Balsalazide
Basiliximab
Benazepril
Benzphetamine
Bepridil
Betaxolol
Bexarotene (5–11%)
Bicalutamide
Bivalirudin
Bortezomib (27%)
Bromocriptine
Buclizine
Bupropion
Buspirone
Calcitonin
Capecitabine
Carbinoxamine
Carmustine
Carteolol
Carvedilol
Caspofungin
Cefaclor

Cefdinir
Cefditoren
Cefpodoxime
Cefprozil
Ceftibuten
Celecoxib
Cetuximab (10%)
Cevimeline
Chlorpromazine
Cidofovir
Cinoxacin
Ciprofloxacin
Citalopram (15%)
Cladribine
Clarithromycin
Clemastine
Clomipramine (>10%)
Clonazepam (>10%)
Clonidine
Clopidogrel
Clorazepate
Clozapine
Corticosteroids
Cyclosporine
Daclizumab
Daptomycin
Darbepoetin alfa
Denileukin
Desipramine
Desmopressin
Dextroamphetamine
Diazepam
Dicyclomine
Didanosine
Dimenhydrinate
Diphenhydramine
Disopyramide
Dofetilide
Donepezil
Doxazosin
Doxorubicin
Duloxetine (10%)
Efavirenz
Emtricitabine (7–16%)

Enfuvirtide (11%)
Enoxaparin
Entacapone
Ephedrine
Epinephrine
Ertapenem
Escitalopram
Estazolam
Estramustine
Etanercept
Etodolac
Exemestane (11%)
Famotidine
Felodipine
Fenofibrate
Fexofenadine
Fludarabine
Flumazenil
Fluoxetine (10–33%)
Fluoxymesterone
Fluphenazine
Flurazepam
Flurbiprofen
Flutamide
Fluvastatin
Fluvoxamine (>10%)
Fondaparinux
Formoterol
Fosinopril
Fosphenytoin
Frovatriptan
Fulvestrant
Galantamine
Gatifloxacin
Gemcitabine
Gemifloxacin
Gemtuzumab (18%)
Glipizide
Glycopyrrolate
Goserelin
Granisetron
Griseofulvin
Guanabenz
Guanfacine

Guarana
Haloperidol
Hepatitis B vaccine
Hyoscyamine
Ibandronate
Ibritumomab
Idebenone
Imatinib (10–13%)
Imipramine
Indapamide
Indinavir
Indomethacin
Influenza vaccines
Interferon alfa-2A (14%)
Interferon beta-1B (24%)
Irinotecan (>10%)
Isoetharine
Isotretinoin
Isradipine
Ivermectin
Ketoprofen
Labetalol
Lamivudine
Lamotrigine
Letrozole
Leuprolide
Levalbuterol
Levamisole
Levetiracetam
Levobetaxolol
Levobunolol
Levodopa
Levofloxacin
Levothyroxine
Linezolid
Liothyronine
Lomefloxacin
Loracarbef
Loratadine
Losartan
Lovastatin
Loxapine
Maprotiline
Meclizine

Meclofenamate
Medroxyprogesterone
Mefenamic acid
Mefloquine
Memantine
Mepenzolate
Mephenytoin
Mephobarbital
Mesalamine
Mesoridazine
Metaxalone
Methadone
Methamphetamine
Methantheline
Methocarbamol
Methoxsalen
Methylphenidate
Methyltestosterone
Methysergide
Metipranolol
Metoclopramide
Metolazone
Metoprolol (>10%)
Metronidazole
Mexiletine
Midodrine
Mifepristone
Modafinil
Montelukast
Moricizine
Morphine
Moxifloxacin
Mycophenolate (41–52%)
Nabumetone
Nadolol (>10%)
Nafarelin
Nalbuphine
Naltrexone (>10%)
Naproxen
Naratriptan
Natalizumab
Nefazodone (>10%)
Nesiritide
Niacin

Nicotine
Nizatidine
Norfloxacin
Nortriptyline
Ofloxacin
Olanzapine (>10%)
Olmesartan
Oseltamivir
Oxaliplatin (11%)
Oxaprozin
Oxcarbazepine
Oxybutynin
Pamidronate
Paramethadione
Paroxetine (>10%)
Peginterferon alfa-2B (23%)
Pegvisomant
Pemetrexed
Pemoline
Penbutolol (>10%)
Pentazocine
Pentobarbital
Pentostatin
Pergolide
Perphenazine
Phenindamine
Phenobarbital
Phentermine
Phenylephrine
Phenytoin
Pindolol (10%)
Pirbuterol
Piroxicam
Pramipexole (>10%)
Pravastatin
Procarbazine (>10%)
Prochlorperazine
Procyclidine
Progestins
Promazine
Promethazine
Propantheline
Propoxyphene
Propranolol (>10%)

Protriptyline
Pseudoephedrine
Pyrimethamine
Quinapril
Raloxifene
Ramipril
Ranitidine
Ribavirin
Rifabutin
Riluzole
Rimantadine
Risperidone (>10%)
Ritonavir
Rituximab
Rivastigmine
Rizatriptan
Rosuvastatin
Sertraline
Sibutramine
Sodium oxybate
Sparfloxacin
Stanozolol
Stavudine
Telithromycin
Teriparatide
Theophylline
Tiagabine
Topiramate
Tranylcypromine
Trioxsalen
Unoprostone
Valganciclovir
Vigabatrin
Zalcitabine
Zaleplon
Zidovudine
Zileuton
Zonisamide

IRRITABILITY
Albuterol
Alprazolam (10–33%)
Alprostadil (<1%)
Amantadine (1–5%)

Aminophylline
Atomoxetine
Bupropion
Capecitabine
Cefpodoxime
Ceftibuten
Chlordiazepoxide
Ciprofloxacin
Clemastine
Clofarabine (11%)
Clonazepam
Clorazepate
Clozapine
Cyclobenzaprine
Cycloserine
Daptomycin
Dextromethorphan
Dicyclomine
Didanosine
Dimenhydrinate
Duloxetine
Efavirenz
Entacapone
Ephedrine
Epinephrine
Ethosuximide
Ethotoin
Etodolac
Felodipine
Flavoxate
Fluoxetine
Fosphenytoin
Fulvestrant
Gabapentin
Glycopyrrolate
Guanabenz
Hepatitis B vaccine
Hydrochlorothiazide
Hydroflumethiazide
Hydroxychloroquine
Ibuprofen
Immune globulin IV
Indomethacin
Interferon alfa-2A (15%)

Isoetharine
Isradipine
Ketoprofen
Lamotrigine
Levetiracetam
Levothyroxine
Lindane
Liothyronine
Loratadine
Meclofenamate
Medroxyprogesterone
Mefenamic acid
Memantine
Mephenytoin
Metaxalone
Methocarbamol
Methsuximide
Methyclothiazide
Metoclopramide
Metronidazole
Montelukast
Naloxone
Naltrexone
Naproxen
Natalizumab
Nicotine
Nitisinone
Nizatidine
Orphenadrine
Oxcarbazepine
Paramethadione
Peginterferon alfa-2B (28%)
Pemetrexed
Pemoline
Pentazocine
Phenindamine
Phenytoin
Phytonadione
Piroxicam
Polythiazide
Primidone
Propoxyphene
Ranitidine
Rasburicase

Reteplase
Ribavirin
Rimantadine
Rizatriptan
Sibutramine
Sirolimus
Sodium oxybate
Streptokinase
Theophylline
Thiabendazole
Topiramate
Trimethadione
Urokinase
Zidovudine
Zonisamide

LACRIMATION
Atomoxetine
Cevimeline
Dextroamphetamine
Flumazenil
Gabapentin
Methamphetamine
Sirolimus
Triptorelin
Vidarabine

LETHAGY
Alosetron
Alprostadil (<1%)
Alprazolam
Anastrozole
Aspirin
Benzonatate
Betaxolol
Clofarabine (11%)
Clonidine
Clozapine
Daptomycin
Dicyclomine
Duloxetine
Epirubicin (1–46%)
Estramustine
Fluphenazine

Glycopyrrolate
Goserelin
Haloperidol
Immune globulin IV
Indapamide
Interferon alfa-2A
Isoniazid
Isotretinoin
Isradipine
Levobetaxolol
Levobunolol
Lidocaine
Lithium
Mesoridazine
Metipranolol
Oxazepam
Pentobarbital
Perphenazine
Phenobarbital
Phenoxybenzamine
Prazepam
Primidone
Promazine
Promethazine
Quazepam
Reteplase
Streptokinase

LIBIDO CHANGED
Aripiprazole
Atomoxetine
Benazepril
Benzphetamine
Bepridil
Bicalutamide
Cabergoline
Chlordiazepoxide (>10%)
Chlorotrianisene
Citalopram
Clofibrate
Clomipramine (>10%)
Clonazepam
Clonidine
Clorazepate

Desipramine
Dextroamphetamine
Disulfiram
Doxazosin
Duloxetine
Ergocalciferol
Escitalopram
Estramustine
Ethionamide
Felodipine
Fenofibrate
Finasteride
Fluoxetine
Fluoxymesterone
Fluphenazine
Flutamide (>10%)
Fluvastatin
Fluvoxamine
Glatiramer
Goserelin (61%)
Guanabenz
Guanethidine
Guanfacine
Haloperidol
Hydrochlorothiazide
Hydroflumethiazide
Hyoscyamine
Imipramine
Interferon beta-1B
Irbesartan
Isradipine
Itraconazole
Ketoconazole
Leuprolide
Lisinopril
Lovastatin
Loxapine
Maprotiline
Mecamylamine
Medroxyprogesterone
Mefloquine
Mepenzolate
Mesoridazine
Methadone

Methamphetamine
Methantheline
Methyclothiazide
Methyldopa
Methyltestosterone
Metoclopramide
Metolazone
Metoprolol
Metronidazole
Mirtazapine
Misoprostol
Moexipril
Molindone
Morphine
Nafarelin (>10%)
Nalbuphine
Naltrexone
Nefazodone
Nelfinavir
Nifedipine
Nortriptyline
Oxazepam
Oxybutynin
Paroxetine
Perindopril
Perphenazine
Phenelzine
Phenoxybenzamine
Phentermine
Pimozide
Polythiazide
Pramipexole
Pravastatin
Prazepam
Primidone
Prochlorperazine
Progestins
Promazine
Promethazine
Propantheline
Protriptyline
Quazepam
Quinapril
Quinethazone

Ramipril
Risperidone
Ropinirole
Sertraline
Sirolimus
Stanozolol
Tamsulosin
Terazosin
Tranylcypromine
Trimipramine
Triptorelin
Venlafaxine

MANIA

Amantadine
Aripiprazole
Atomoxetine
Carbamazepine
Cevimeline
Ciprofloxacin
Clarithromycin
Corticosteroids
Desipramine
Dicyclomine
Felbamate
Fluvoxamine
Glatiramer
Glycopyrrolate
Imipramine
Lamotrigine
Modafinil
Paroxetine
Phenelzine
Procarbazine (>10%)
Propantheline
Zalcitabine

MOOD CHANGES

Atomoxetine
Capecitabine
Corticosteroids
Cycloserine
Dihydrotachysterol
Disulfiram

Dronabinol (>10%)
Efavirenz
Enflurane
Ergocalciferol
Ethacrynic acid
Ethionamide
Ethosuximide
Felbamate
Flumazenil
Fluoxetine
Flurbiprofen
Fluvoxamine
Fondaparinux
Fosamprenavir
Furosemide
Galantamine
Ganciclovir
Glatiramer
Goserelin
Halothane
Hydrochlorothiazide
Hydroflumethiazide
Hydroxychloroquine
Hydroxyurea
Ibandronate
Imatinib
Indapamide
Interferon beta-1A
Interferon beta-1B
Isoflurane
Isoniazid
Itraconazole
Ketamine
Ketoconazole
Labetalol
Leuprolide
Levetiracetam
Levothyroxine
Liothyronine
Medroxyprogesterone
Mefloquine
Methohexital
Methoxyflurane
Methsuximide

Methyclothiazide
Metoprolol
Mirtazapine
Modafinil
Nadolol
Nafarelin (>10%)
Nalidixic acid
Naratriptan
Nefazodone
Nifedipine
Nitisinone
Nitrofurantoin
Olanzapine
Pamidronate
Paramethadione
Peginterferon alfa-2B (28%)
Pemetrexed
Penbutolol
Pindolol
Polythiazide
Pramipexole
Primidone
Procyclidine
Propofol
Propranolol
Ribavirin
Rifampin
Riluzole
Risperidone
Ritonavir
Sibutramine
Sirolimus
Telithromycin
Tiagabine
Tinidazole
Tizanidine
Topiramate
Torsemide
Travoprost
Trimetrexate
Triptorelin
Vigabatrin
Zalcitabine
Zoledronic acid

NERVOUSNESS

Acitretin (<1%)
Acyclovir
Albuterol
Alemtuzumab
Allopurinol IV
Almotriptan
Alprazolam (4%)
Amantadine (1–5%)
Aminophylline
Amlodipine
Amoxapine
Amoxicillin
Amphotericin B
Anagrelide
Anastrozole
Apraclonidine
Aprotinin
Aripiprazole
Arsenic
Asparaginase
Aspirin
Azithromycin
Balsalazide
Basiliximab
Benazepril
Benztropine
Bepridil
Bexarotene
Bicalutamide
Biperiden
Bivalirudin
Bortezomib
Bromocriptine
Bupropion
Buspirone
Cabergoline
Calcitonin
Captopril
Carbamazepine
Carbinoxamine
Carteolol
Carvedilol
Cefaclor

Cefditoren
Ceftibuten
Cefpodoxime
Cefprozil
Celecoxib
Cephalexin
Chlorambucil
Cimetidine
Citalopram
Clemastine
Clomiphene
Clomipramine (>10%)
Clonazepam (>10%)
Clonidine
Clorazepate
Clozapine
Cocaine
Codeine
Corticosteroids
Cyanocobalamin
Cyclobenzaprine
Cyclophosphamide
Cycloserine
Cyclosporine
Cyproheptadine
Danazol
Dantrolene
Dapsone
Daptomycin
Denileukin (11%)
Desflurane
Desipramine
Desmopressin
Dextroamphetamine
Dextromethorphan
Dicloxacillin
Dicumarol
Dicyclomine
Dihydroergotamine
Diltiazem
Dimenhydrinate
Diphenhydramine
Diphenoxylate
Disopyramide

Doxazosin
Dronabinol
Duloxetine
Efavirenz
Entacapone
Ephedrine
Epinephrine
Eplerenone
Ertapenem
Esmolol
Ethotoin
Ethchlorvynol
Ethionamide
Etodolac
Felbamate
Felodipine
Fenofibrate
Fentanyl
Fexofenadine
Flavoxate
Fludarabine
Flumazenil
Fluoxetine (8–14%)
Fluphenazine
Flurazepam
Flurbiprofen
Fluvoxamine (>10%)
Fomepizole
Fosinopril
Fosphenytoin
Frovatriptan
Fulvestrant
Gabapentin
Gadodiamide
Ganciclovir
Gatifloxacin
Gemifloxacin
Glatiramer
Glimepiride
Glipizide
Glyburide
Glycopyrrolate
Goserelin
Granisetron

Guanabenz
Haloperidol
Hepatitis B vaccine
Hydrocodone
Hydroxychloroquine
Hydroxyurea
Hydroxyzine
Hyoscyamine
Ibandronate
Ibuprofen
Ifosfamide
Imipramine
Indapamide
Indomethacin
Insulin
Interferon beta-1B
Ipratropium
Irbesartan
Isocarboxazid
Isoetharine
Isoproterenol
Isotretinoin
Isradipine
Ketoprofen
Labetalol
Lamotrigine
Lansoprazole
Letrozole
Leuprolide
Levalbuterol
Levamisole
Levetiracetam
Levodopa
Levofloxacin
Levothyroxine
Lidocaine
Lindane
Liothyronine
Lomefloxacin
Loracarbef
Loratadine
Loxapine
Maprotiline
Meclizine
Meclofenamate
Medroxyprogesterone
Mefenamic acid
Mefloquine
Meloxicam
Memantine
Mepenzolate
Meperidine
Mephenytoin
Mephobarbital
Mesoridazine
Methadone
Methamphetamine
Methantheline
Methazolamide
Methicillin
Methoxsalen
Methylphenidate
Metolazone
Metoprolol
Mexiletine
Mezlocillin
Midazolam
Midodrine
Mirtazapine
Modafinil
Montelukast
Morphine
Moxifloxacin
Mycophenolate
Nabumetone
Nadolol
Nafcillin
Nalbuphine
Naltrexone (>10%)
Naproxen
Nateglinide
Nefazodone (>10%)
Nicardipine
Nicotine
Nifedipine
Nitisinone
Nizatidine
Norfloxacin

Nortriptyline
Ofloxacin
Olanzapine (>10%)
Orphenadrine
Oxacillin
Oxaprozin
Oxcarbazepine
Oxybutynin
Oxycodone
Palivizumab
Pamidronate
Paroxetine
Peginterferon alfa-2B
Pegvisomant
Pemoline
Penbutolol
Penicillamine
Penicillins
Pentamidine
Pentazocine
Pentobarbital
Pentostatin
Pergolide
Perindopril
Perphenazine
Phenelzine
Phenindamine
Phenobarbital
Phenytoin
Physostigmine
Pilocarpine
Pindolol
Piperacillin
Pirbuterol (>10%)
Piroxicam
Prazosin
Procarbazine (>10%)
Prochlorperazine
Progestins
Promazine
Promethazine
Propantheline
Propofol
Propoxyphene
Propranolol
Protriptyline
Pseudoephedrine
Quetiapine (>10%)
Quinine
Ramipril
Ranitidine
Rasburicase
Repaglinide
Reserpine
Reteplase
Rimantadine
Risperidone (>10%)
Ritodrine
Rituximab
Rizatriptan
Rosiglitazone
Salmeterol
Sertraline
Sibutramine
Sodium oxybate
Sparfloxacin
Streptokinase
Sulindac
Telithromycin
Terbutaline
Tiagabine
Tinzaparin
Tizanidine
Tolmetin
Topiramate
Travoprost
Trazodone
Trioxsalen
Urokinase
Valdecoxib
Valganciclovir
Venlafaxine
Vigabatrin
Voriconazole
Zalcitabine
Zidovudine
Zileuton
Ziprasidone

Zolmitriptan
Zonisamide

NEUROSIS
Efavirenz
Misoprostol

NEUROTOXICITY
Altretamine (21%)
Amikacin
Cladribine
Kanamycin
Lomustine
Neomycin
Nimodipine
Streptomycin

NIGHTMARES
Albuterol
Alprazolam (1–10%)
Amitriptyline
Atenolol
Bromocriptine
Bupropion
Carteolol
Cefpodoxime
Chloral hydrate
Ciprofloxacin
Clarithromycin
Clonidine
Clozapine
Codeine
Cycloserine
Dimenhydrinate
Dronabinol
Duloxetine
Enflurane
Ethosuximide
Fexofenadine
Fluoxetine
Glimepiride
Glipizide
Glyburide
Halothane

Hydrocodone
Hydroxychloroquine
Imipramine
Insulin
Isoetharine
Isoflurane
Ketamine
Labetalol
Levamisole
Levodopa
Meperidine
Mephenytoin
Mephobarbital
Metformin
Methadone
Methohexital
Methoxyflurane
Methsuximide
Methyldopa
Methysergide
Metoprolol
Morphine
Nabumetone
Nalbuphine
Nateglinide
Nortriptyline
Oxaprozin
Oxycodone
Penbutolol
Pentazocine
Pentobarbital
Phenobarbital
Phenytoin
Pindolol
Procarbazine (>10%)
Propofol
Propoxyphene
Propranolol
Protriptyline
Repaglinide
Reserpine
Rosiglitazone
Secobarbital
Selegiline

Tiagabine
Tranylcypromine
Trazodone
Trimipramine

NYSTAGMUS

Acetazolamide
Acetylcysteine
Albuterol
Alprazolam (41–77%)
Amoxapine
Apomorphine
Atenolol
Baclofen (10–63%)
Bepridil
Betaxolol
Biperiden
Botulinum toxin (a & b)
Bromocriptine
Buclizine
Buspirone (10%)
Candesartan
Carbamazepine
Carbinoxamine
Carisoprodol
Chloral hydrate
Chlordiazepoxide (>10%)
Chlorpromazine
Chlorzoxazone
Cimetidine
Citalopram
Clofazimine
Clomipramine (>10%)
Clonazepam (>10%)
Clonidine (35%)
Clorazepate
Clozapine (>10%)
Codeine (>10%)
Colestipol
Cyclobenzaprine (29–39%)
Cycloserine
Cyproheptadine (>10%)
Dantrolene
Desipramine

Dextromethorphan
Diazepam
Dihydroergotamine
Dihydrotachysterol
Dimenhydrinate
Diphenhydramine
Diphenoxylate
Disopyramide
Disulfiram
Dolasetron
Doxepin (topical: 22%)
Doxercalciferol
Dronabinol (48%)
Droperidol
Edrophonium
Eletriptan
Emtricitabine
Enflurane
Entacapone
Ergocalciferol
Ertapenem
Escitalopram
Estazolam
Etanercept
Ethchlorvynol
Ethionamide
Ethosuximide
Ethotoin
Etodolac
Famotidine
Fentanyl
Fexofenadine
Flavoxate
Flucytosine
Fluoxetine
Fluphenazine
Flurazepam
Flurbiprofen
Flutamide
Fluvoxamine
Fosfomycin
Fosphenytoin (<10%)
Frovatriptan
Gabapentin

Gadodiamide
Galantamine
Gemcitabine
Glimepiride
Glipizide
Glyburide
Glycopyrrolate
Granisetron
Guanfacine
Haloperidol
Halothane
Hydrocodone (>10%)
Hydroxychloroquine
Hydroxyzine
Hyoscyamine
Ibuprofen
Imipramine
Immune globulin IV
Indapamide
Indomethacin
Insulin
Isocarboxazid
Isoetharine
Isoflurane
Isotretinoin
Ketamine
Ketoprofen
Ketorolac
Lamotrigine
Levobetaxolol
Levobunolol
Lidocaine
Lithium
Loperamide
Loracarbef
Loxapine
Mafenide
Maprotiline
Mecamylamine
Meclizine
Meclofenamate
Mefenamic acid
Mefloquine
Meloxicam

Memantine
Mepenzolate
Meperidine (>10%)
Mephenytoin (<10%)
Meprobamate
Mesoridazine
Metaxalone
Metformin
Methadone
Methamphetamine
Methantheline
Methazolamide
Methimazole
Methocarbamol
Methoxyflurane
Methsuximide
Methyldopa
Methylphenidate
Metoclopramide
Metolazone
Metoprolol (>10%)
Midazolam
Midodrine
Mirtazapine
Misoprostol
Mitotane
Molindone
Morphine (48%)
Nadolol (>10%)
Nalbuphine (>10%)
Nalidixic acid
Naproxen
Naratriptan
Natalizumab
Nateglinide
Nefazodone (>10%)
Nelfinavir
Nesiritide
Nitisinone
Nitrofurantoin
Nizatidine
Nortriptyline
Olsalazine
Omeprazole

Orphenadrine
Oxaprozin
Oxazepam
Oxcarbazepine (7–26%)
Oxybutynin
Oxycodone (>10%)
Pamidronate
Pantoprazole
Papaverine
Paramethadione
Paroxetine
Peginterferon alfa-2B
Penbutolol (>10%)
Penicillins
Pentagastrin
Pentamidine
Pentazocine
Pentobarbital
Perphenazine
Phenelzine
Phenobarbital
Phenoxybenzamine
Phenytoin
Pindolol (>10%)
Plicamycin
Prazepam
Praziquantel
Prazosin
Primidone
Procarbazine (>10%)
Prochlorperazine
Procyclidine
Progestins
Promazine
Promethazine
Propantheline
Propofol
Propoxyphene
Propranolol
Propylthiouracil
Protriptyline
Pseudoephedrine
Quazepam
Ranitidine

Repaglinide
Reserpine
Reteplase
Riluzole
Risperidone
Rizatriptan
Ropinirole
Salsalate
Scopolamine
Secobarbital
Sertraline
Sibutramine
Sirolimus
Solifenacin
Sparfloxacin
Spironolactone
Streptokinase
Sufentanil
Sumatriptan
Tamsulosin
Telithromycin
Temazepam
Terazosin
Terbutaline
Thalidomide
Thiabendazole
Thiopental
Thioridazine
Thiothixene
Tiagabine
Tizanidine
Topiramate
Tramadol
Tranylcypromine
Triazolam
Trifluoperazine
Trihexyphenidyl
Trimeprazine
Trimethadione
Trimethobenzamide
Trimipramine
Tripelennamine
Triprolidine
Trovafloxacin

Valproic acid
Vancomycin
Vasopressin
Vigabatrin
Zaleplon
Zidovudine
Ziprasidone
Zolmitriptan
Zolpidem
Zonisamide

PANIC
Citalopram
Diethylpropion
Dronabinol
Flumazenil
Gatifloxacin
Levofloxacin
Lomefloxacin
Losartan
Mazindol
Mefloquine
Moxifloxacin
Norfloxacin
Ofloxacin
Phendimetrazine
Phentermine

PARANOIA
Aldesleukin (>10%)
Amantadine
Aripiprazole
Bromocriptine
Carmustine
Cevimeline
Citalopram
Cocaine
Delavirdine
Dextroamphetamine
Dicyclomine
Doxazosin
Efavirenz
Flumazenil
Fluoxetine

Fluoxymesterone
Galantamine
Gatifloxacin
Glycopyrrolate
Levamisole
Levofloxacin
Lomefloxacin
Mefloquine
Methamphetamine
Methyltestosterone
Moxifloxacin
Naltrexone
Nifedipine
Norfloxacin
Ofloxacin
Paroxetine
Pramipexole
Ribavirin
Triptorelin
Zalcitabine

PRIAPISM
Androstenedione
Anisindione
Aripiprazole
Bupropion
Chlorpromazine
Citalopram
Clozapine
Cocaine
Codeine
Dicumarol
Doxazosin
Droperidol
Fluoxetine
Fluoxymesterone (>10%)
Fluphenazine
Fluvoxamine
Gabapentin
Glatiramer
Guanfacine
Haloperidol
Hydrocodone
Hydroxyzine

Labetalol
Levodopa
Loxapine
MDMA
Meperidine
Mesoridazine
Methadone
Methyltestosterone (>10%)
Metoprolol
Molindone
Morphine
Nadolol
Nalbuphine
Nefazodone
Olanzapine
Oxcarbazepine
Oxycodone
Papaverine (11%)
Paroxetine
Penbutolol
Pentazocine
Pergolide
Perphenazine
Phenelzine
Phenoxybenzamine
Pindolol
Prazosin
Prochlorperazine
Promazine
Promethazine
Propoxyphene
Propranolol
Quetiapine
Risperidone (<10%)
Sildenafil
Stanozolol
Tadalafil
Tamsulosin
Terazosin
Trazodone
Vardenafil
Ziprasidone

PSYCHOSIS
Acyclovir (<1%)
Aldesleukin (1%)
Amantadine (<1%)
Aripiprazole
Benzphetamine
Benztropine
Bromocriptine
Bupropion
Chloroquine
Chlorpromazine
Cimetidine
Citalopram
Clarithromycin
Cocaine
Corticosteroids
Cyclobenzaprine
Cycloserine
Desipramine
Disopyramide
Disulfiram
Enalapril
Felbamate
Flucytosine
Gatifloxacin
Hydroxychloroquine
Ifosfamide
Indomethacin
Interferon alfa-2A
Interferon beta-1B
Isoniazid
Isotretinoin
Levetiracetam
Levofloxacin
Lidocaine
Lomefloxacin
Losartan
Mefloquine
Methamphetamine
Methylphenidate
Mexiletine
Modafinil
Moxifloxacin
Mycophenolate

Nitrofurantoin
Nizatidine
Norfloxacin
Nortriptyline
Ofloxacin
Oxcarbazepine
Pamidronate
Penicillamine
Pergolide
Phentermine
Propantheline
Propranolol
Protriptyline
Quinidine
Ranitidine
Risperidone
Rivastigmine
Rizatriptan
Sparfloxacin
Trazodone
Vigabatrin
Zalcitabine

SCHIZOPHRENIC REACTION
Aripiprazole

SEDATION
Chloral hydrate
Clemastine
Clonidine
Cyproheptadine
Diphenhydramine
Dronabinol (53%)
Droperidol
Fentanyl
Flucytosine
Loperamide
Lorazepam
Methadone
Methocarbamol
Molindone
Morphine
Nalbuphine
Oxaprozin

Oxazepam
Propoxyphene
Quazepam
Risperidone
Sufentanil

SHOCK
Alprostadil (<1%)
Indomethacin
Interferon beta-1B
Isosorbide dinitrate
Isosorbide mononitrate
Meloxicam
Moxifloxacin
Nitroglycerin
Ondansetron
Oxaprozin
Pentazocine
Phenoxybenzamine
Propoxyphene
Quinapril
Quinupristin/Dalfopristin
Ramipril

SLEEP DISTURBANCE
Abarelix (44%)
Amiodarone
Atomoxetine
Carvedilol
Cefaclor
Cefuroxime
Clomipramine
Clonazepam
Disopyramide
Duloxetine
Orlistat
Perindopril
Phenelzine
Quinidine
Telithromycin
Tinidazole
Tizanidine
Tolcapone
Trazodone

Trimipramine
Triptorelin
Valganciclovir
Zolmitriptan

SOMNAMBULISM
Sodium oxybate

SOMNOLENCE
Acamprosate
Acitretin (1–10%)
Acyclovir (<1%)
Aldesleukin (22%)
Alemtuzumab (5%)
Almotriptan (>1%)
Amantadine (1–5%)
Amifostine
Amiloride
Amlodipine
Amphotericin B
Anagrelide
Anastrozole
Apomorphine
Apraclonidine
Aripiprazole
Arsenic
Asparaginase
Atomoxetine
Azithromycin
Balsalazide
Benazepril
Bicalutamide
Brimonidine
Cabergoline
Candesartan
Captopril
Carbamazepine (>10%)
Carmustine (11%)
Carvedilol
Cefaclor
Cefdinir
Cefditoren
Cefprozil
Cefuroxime

Celecoxib
Cetirizine (14%)
Cevimeline
Cimetidine
Citalopram (18%)
Clemastine
Clofarabine (10%)
Cytarabine
Desloratadine
Desmopressin
Dextroamphetamine
Dicyclomine
Dihydroergotamine
Donepezil
Doxazosin
Doxorubicin
Duloxetine (10%)
Efavirenz
Eprosartan
Ertapenem
Esmolol
Famciclovir
Felodipine
Fenofibrate
Fenoprofen (9–15%)
Finasteride
Flecainide
Fludarabine (30%)
Fluorouracil
Fluoxetine (5–17%)
Flurbiprofen
Fluvoxamine (>10%)
Fosfomycin
Fosphenytoin (<10%)
Gabapentin (20%)
Galantamine
Gatifloxacin
Gemcitabine (11%)
Gemifloxacin
Glycopyrrolate
Goserelin
Granisetron
Ifosfamide
Imipenem/Cilastatin

Indomethacin
Interferon alfa-2A
Interferon beta-1A
Isradipine
Itraconazole
Ivermectin
Ketoconazole
Ketoprofen
Lamotrigine (14%)
Letrozole
Leuprolide
Levetiracetam (15%)
Levofloxacin
Lomefloxacin
Loracarbef
Loratadine
Meclofenamate
Medroxyprogesterone
Mefenamic acid
Mefloquine
Meloxicam
Memantine
Mephenytoin (<10%)
Mephobarbital
Midodrine
Mirtazapine (54%)
Modafinil
Moxifloxacin
Mycophenolate
Nabumetone
Naltrexone
Nelfinavir
Nesiritide
Nevirapine
Nicardipine
Nicotine
Nifedipine
Nisoldipine
Nitisinone
Nizatidine
Norfloxacin
Ofloxacin
Olanzapine (>10%)
Omeprazole

Oxaprozin
Oxcarbazepine (20–36%)
Oxybutynin (12%)
Oxycodone (>10%)
Pamidronate
Paroxetine
Pentazocine (>10%)
Pentobarbital
Pentostatin
Pergolide (10%)
Phenindamine
Phenobarbital
Phenytoin
Pilocarpine
Pramipexole (>10%)
Propoxyphene (>10%)
Quetiapine (>10%)
Quinapril
Ramipril
Ranitidine
Risperidone
Ritonavir
Rituximab
Rivastigmine
Ropinirole (40%)
Sermorelin
Thalidomide
Tinidazole
Tolcapone
Tripelennamine
Venlafaxine
Zalcitabine
Zonisamide

STUPOR
Aldesleukin (1%)
Alprazolam (>10%)
Amantadine
Amitriptyline
Aripiprazole
Carbamazepine
Carmustine
Cefepime
Citalopram

Daptomycin
Dicyclomine
Ertapenem
Felbamate
Flecainide
Fluoxetine
Fosphenytoin
Glatiramer
Glycopyrrolate
Lithium
Mephenytoin
Oxcarbazepine
Phenytoin
Rasburicase
Reteplase
Streptokinase
Zalcitabine

SUICIDAL IDEATION (SUICIDE)
Acamprosate
Amantadine (<1%)
Aripiprazole
Cetirizine
Citalopram
Clofazimine
Cycloserine
Duloxetine
Efavirenz
Felbamate
Glatiramer
Interferon alfa-2A (>15%)
Interferon beta-1A
Interferon beta-1B
Isotretinoin
Lamotrigine
Mefloquine
Metoclopramide
Naltrexone
Natalizumab
Nelfinavir
Peginterferon alfa-2B
Thimerosal
Zalcitabine

SYNCOPE
Abarelix
Acamprosate
Alemtuzumab
Alfuzosin (<1%)
Almotriptan (<1%)
Alprazolam (3–4%)
Amlodipine
Amoxapine
Anagrelide
Azithromycin
Baclofen
Benazepril
Bepridil
Bevacizumab
Bexarotene
Bicalutamide
Bivalirudin
Botulinum toxin (a & b)
Bretylium
Bromocriptine
Bupropion
Cabergoline
Capecitabine
Captopril
Carbamazepine
Carbinoxamine
Carisoprodol
Carteolol
Carvedilol
Cefpodoxime
Celecoxib
Cetirizine
Cevimeline
Chlorpromazine
Ciprofloxacin
Citalopram
Clonidine
Clopidogrel
Clozapine
Cyclobenzaprine
Cytarabine
Daptomycin
Darbepoetin alfa

Delavirdine
Denileukin
Dextroamphetamine
Dicloxacillin
Dicumarol
Dicyclomine
Diethylpropion
Diflunisal
Digoxin
Diltiazem
Dinoprostone
Dipyridamole
Disopyramide
Dobutamine
Docetaxel
Dofetilide
Domperidone
Donepezil
Doxazosin
Dronabinol
Edrophonium
Efavirenz
Enalapril
Enflurane
Enoxaparin
Entacapone
Epoetin alfa
Eprosartan
Ertapenem
Erythromycin
Estrogens
Ethchlorvynol
Etodolac
Felodipine
Fentanyl
Flecainide
Fluoxetine
Fluphenazine
Flurbiprofen
Flutamide
Foscarnet
Fosinopril
Fosphenytoin
Frovatriptan

Fulvestrant
Gadodiamide
Galantamine
Gatifloxacin
Gemfibrozil
Gemtuzumab
Glatiramer
Glipizide
Granisetron
Granulocyte colony-stimulating factor (GCSF)
Guanadrel
Guanethidine
Guanfacine
Haloperidol
Halothane
Hepatitis B vaccine
Hyaluronic acid
Hydroxyurea
Hydroxyzine
Hyoscyamine
Ibandronate
Ibritumomab
Ibuprofen
Ifosfamide
Imatinib (11–13%)
Imiglucerase
Imipenem/Cilastatin
Indomethacin
Interferon alfa-2A
Interferon beta-1B
Irbesartan
Irinotecan
Isosorbide dinitrate
Isosorbide mononitrate
Isoxsuprine
Ketamine
Labetalol
Laronidase
Leflunomide
Letrozole
Leuprolide
Levalbuterol
Levodopa

Levofloxacin
Lithium
Lomefloxacin
Loratadine
Losartan
Loxapine
Maprotiline
Medroxyprogesterone
Meloxicam
Mepenzolate
Mephenytoin
Mephobarbital
Meprobamate
Mesoridazine
Metaxalone
Methamphetamine
Methantheline
Methicillin
Methocarbamol
Methohexital
Methoxyflurane
Metolazone
Metoprolol
Mexiletine
Mezlocillin
Midodrine
Mifepristone
Moexipril
Moricizine
Moxifloxacin
Nabumetone
Nadolol
Nafcillin
Naproxen
Naratriptan
Natalizumab
Nefazodone
Nelfinavir
Nesiritide
Niacin
Nicardipine
Nifedipine
Nisoldipine
Nitisinone

Nitroglycerin
Norfloxacin
Ofloxacin
Orphenadrine
Oxaprozin
Oxcarbazepine
Oxybutynin
Oxycodone
Palonosetron
Pamidronate
Pantoprazole
Paroxetine
Penbutolol
Penicillins
Pentagastrin
Pentazocine
Pentobarbital
Pergolide
Perindopril
Perphenazine
Phendimetrazine
Phenindamine
Phenobarbital
Phenoxybenzamine
Phentermine
Phenytoin
Phytonadione
Pilocarpine
Pimozide
Pindolol
Piperacillin
Piroxicam
Pramipexole
Prazepam
Prazosin
Procarbazine
Prochlorperazine
Promazine
Promethazine
Propantheline
Propofol
Propoxyphene
Propranolol
Quazepam

Quetiapine
Quinapril
Quinethazone
Quinidine
Quinine
Quinupristin/Dalfopristin
Rabeprazole
Ramipril
Reteplase
Ritonavir
Rivastigmine
Rizatriptan
Ropinirole (12%)
Rosuvastatin
Sildenafil
Sirolimus
Streptokinase
Tegaserod
Telithromycin
Telmisartan

Terazosin
Teriparatide
Thioguanine
Timolol
Tinidazole
Tinzaparin
Tizanidine
Trandolapril
Travoprost
Trazodone
Treprostinil
Trichlormethiazide
Vardenafil
Vasopressin
Verapamil
Zanamivir
Zoledronic acid
Zolmitriptan